# Colonial Modernities

T0174066

The subject of medicalisation of childbirth in colonial India has so far been identified with three major themes: the attempt to reform or 'sanitise' the site of birthing practices, establishing lying-in hospitals and replacing traditional birth attendants with trained midwives and qualified female doctors.

This book, part of the series *The Social History of Health and Medicine in South Asia*, looks at the interactions between childbirth and midwifery practices and colonial modernities. Taking eastern India as a case study and related research from other areas, with hard empirical data from local government bodies, municipal corporations and district boards, it goes beyond the conventional narrative to show how the late nineteenth-century initiatives to reform birthing practices were essentially a modernist response of the western-educated colonised middle class to the colonial critique of Indian sociocultural codes. It provides a perceptive historical analysis of how institutionalisation of midwifery was shaped by the debates on the women's question, nationalism and colonial public health policies, all intersecting in the interwar years. The study traces the beginning of medicalisation of childbirth, the professionalisation of obstetrics, the agency of male doctors, inclusion of midwifery as an academic subject in medical colleges and consequences of maternal care and infant welfare.

This book will greatly interest scholars and researchers in history, social medicine, public policy, gender studies and South Asian studies.

**Ambalika Guha** is an independent researcher based in Kolkata, India. She completed her education at Presidency College, University of Calcutta, Kolkata, India, and Victoria University of Wellington, New Zealand. She is also a member of the New Zealand Asia Society.

# The Social History of Health and Medicine in South Asia

Series editors:

Biswamoy Pati
*Department of History, University of Delhi, India*
Mark Harrison
*Director of the Wellcome Unit for the History of Medicine and Professor of the History of Medicine, University of Oxford, UK*

Since the late 1990s, health and medicine have emerged as major concerns in South Asian history. The Social History of Health and Medicine in South Asia series aims to foster a new wave of interdisciplinary research and scholarship that transcends conventional boundaries. It welcomes proposals for monographs, edited collections and anthologies which offer fresh perspectives, innovative analytical frameworks and comparative assessments. The series embraces diverse aspects of health and healing in colonial and postcolonial contexts.

Books in this series

Colonial Modernities
Midwifery in Bengal, c.1860–1947
*Ambalika Guha*

Society, Medicine and Politics in Colonial India
*Edited by Biswamoy Pati and Mark Harrison*

# Colonial Modernities
## Midwifery in Bengal, c.1860–1947

Ambalika Guha

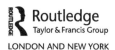
LONDON AND NEW YORK

First published 2018
by Routledge
2 Park Square, Milton Park, Abingdon, Oxon OX14 4RN

and by Routledge
605 Third Avenue, New York, NY 10017

First issued in paperback 2020

*Routledge is an imprint of the Taylor & Francis Group, an informa business*

*British Library Cataloguing-in-Publication Data*
A catalogue record for this book is available from the British Library

*Library of Congress Cataloging-in-Publication Data*
A catalog record has been requested for this book

ISBN 13: 978-0-367-73606-4 (pbk)
ISBN 13: 978-1-138-22191-8 (hbk)

Typeset in Sabon
by Apex CoVantage, LLC

To my parents

# Contents

# Preface

In colonial India, medicalisation of childbirth has been historically perceived as an attempt to 'sanitise' the *zenana* (secluded quarters of a respectable household inhabited by women) as the chief site of birthing practices and to replace the *dhais* (traditional birth attendants) with trained midwives and qualified female doctors. This book takes a broader view of the subject but, in doing so, focuses on Bengal as the geographical area of study. It has argued that medicalisation of childbirth in Bengal was preceded by the reconstitution of midwifery as an academic subject and a medical discipline at the Calcutta Medical College. The consequence was the gradual ascendancy of professionalised obstetrics that prioritised research, surgical intervention and 'surveillance' over women's bodies. The study also shows how the medicalisation of childbirth was sustained and nurtured by the reformist and nationalist discourses of the middle-class Bengalis in the late nineteenth and early twentieth centuries.

The study begins from the 1860s when the earliest scientific essays on childbirth and pregnancy began to appear in Bengali women's magazines such as *Bamabodhini Patrika*. It ends in the 1940s, when nationalism profoundly influenced the professionalisation of obstetrics – midwifery being perceived as the keystone in a nation's progress.

Bengal being the earliest seat of British power in India was also the first to experience contact with the western civilisation, culture and thought. It also had the most elaborate medical establishment along western medical lines since the foundation of the Calcutta Medical College in 1835. It is argued in the extant literature that unlike the West where professionalised obstetrics was characterised as essentially a male domain, the evolving professional domain of obstetrics in Bengal was dominated by female doctors alone. Questioning that argument, the study demonstrates that the domain of obstetrics in Bengal was since the 1880s shared by both female and male doctors, although the role of the latter was more pedagogic and ideological than being directly interventionist. Together they contributed to the evolution of a new medical discourse on childbirth in colonial Bengal.

The study shows how the late-nineteenth-century initiatives to reform birthing practices were essentially a modernist response of the western-educated colonised middle class to the colonial critique of Indian sociocultural codes that also included an explicit reference to the 'low' status of Bengali women. Reforming midwifery constituted one of the ways of modernising the middle-class women as mothers. In the twentieth century, the argument for medicalisation was further driven by nationalist recognition of family and health as important elements of the nation-building process. It also drew sustenance from international movements, such as the global eugenic discourse on the centrality of 'racial regeneration' in national development, and the maternal and infant welfare movement in England and elsewhere in the interwar years. The study provides a historical analysis of how institutionalisation of midwifery was shaped by the debates on women's question, nationalism and colonial public health policies, all intersecting with each other in Bengal in the interwar years.

The study has drawn upon a number of Bengali women's magazines, popular health magazines and professional medical journals in English and Bengali that represent both nationalist and official viewpoints on the medicalisation of childbirth and maternal and infant health. It has also used annual reports of the medical institutions to chart the history of institutionalisation of midwifery and draws upon archival sources – the medical and educational proceedings in particular – in the West Bengal State Archives and the National Archives of India.

# Acknowledgements

This book is based on my doctoral research which I pursued at the Victoria University of Wellington, New Zealand. In the course of writing this book, I have incurred a number of debts. My foremost gratitude is to my supervisors, Professor Sekhar Bandyopadhyay and Professor Charlotte Macdonald, for their constant encouragement and support. Their perceptive comments and painstaking correction of the drafts of my chapters helped me sharpen the focus of my study and give it a better shape. I am also grateful to the other faculty members of the History Programme for critically commenting on my work during the two seminar presentations that I made in the course of my research. I am particularly indebted to Dr Steve Behrendt and Dr Giacomo Lichtner for sharing useful tips on enhancing the quality of research during the weekly students' seminar. I acknowledge my debt to our department librarian Justin Cargill for his untiring support and promptness in answering the most trivial queries even while I was in India for my research trip.

My deepest gratitude is to my teachers at Presidency College, Kolkata, Professor Rajat Kanta Ray and Subhash Ranjan Chakrabarty, for instilling in me an enduring love for history.

I owe my interest in the history of medicine to the meaningful conversations with Dr Rajsekhar Basu, who was my teacher and mentor at the University of Calcutta. Dr Basu introduced me to the vast historical and anthropological literature on the subject. I am greatly indebted to Dr Arabinda Samanta, who suggested that I explore the arena of women's reproductive health. I have gained immensely from the erudition of my teachers at Calcutta University, Professor Hari S. Vasudevan, Professor Suranjan Das, Professor Arun Bandopadhyay, Professor Bhaskar Chakravarty, Professor Amit Dey, Professor Suparna Gooptu and Dr Sanjukta Dasgupta, who have influenced me in myriad ways. The late Dr Krishna Soman of the Institute for

Development Studies, Kolkata, shared her research experience with me and took pain to go through my proposal, adding valuable insights to it. I would also express my gratitude towards Dr Supriya Guha for kindly agreeing to read and comment on my research proposal even though we never met in person.

This book would not have been possible without the enthusiasm of Dr Jane Buckingham of the University of Canterbury, who was not only my examiner but turned out to be a friend and a source of inspiration. Jane's encouragement prodded me to embrace the challenging task of writing a book. Her critical insight and extremely valuable comments helped me arrive at a more nuanced understanding of my subject. I am also indebted to Professor Sanjoy Bhattacharya, my other examiner, for suggesting more thought-provoking ways of approaching the subject.

I am fortunate to have come in touch with Professor Biswamoy Pati, who took interest in my work. Professor Pati's encouragement and promptness in answering my ceaseless queries with remarkable ease not only amazed me but also instilled confidence in me to embrace the task of writing this book with greater zeal than ever.

I also take this opportunity to thank Professor Tanika Sarkar for reading one of my chapters and providing meaningful suggestions in the course of the postgraduate workshop that I attended at the 21st New Zealand Asia Conference in Christchurch.

The initial years of my research would have been impossible without the generous support of the staff of National Library, Kolkata, who helped me access rare and brittle documents, including the nineteenth-century medical journals and reproductive pamphlets. I would thank, in particular, Ashim Mukherjee, Sunita Arora and Uttam Malakar for allowing me to photograph brittle books and journals. The staff members of the Annexe building of the National Library kindly permitted me to procure photocopies of materials in the shortest possible time. Their support and friendly behaviour made research an enjoyable experience at the library.

Thanks are due to Bidisha Chakraborty and Madhuri Banik of the West Bengal State Archives for helping me procure important nineteenth-century government files related to my research and also suggesting new files. I would also like to thank the staff of Bangiya Sahitya Parishad, the National Archives of India, the Nehru Memorial Museum and Library, New Delhi, and the Margaret Cousins Library of the All India Women's Conference for their timely support and help.

I do not have enough words to thank my friend and archivist Kamalika Mukherjee of the Centre for Studies in Social Sciences

(CSSSC), Kolkata, for generously allowing me to consult their brilliant archives at the shortest possible notice and providing me with photocopies of valuable documents.

I have thoroughly enjoyed the intellectual company of my friends in New Zealand, especially Ben Kingbury and Sabbaq Ahmed. I consider myself fortunate to have friends like Subhashri Ghosh, Bidisha Dasgupta, Ratnabir Guha and Ambuj Thakur, who have been my constant source of inspiration and strength.

Thanks are due to Eshita, my dearest friend whose affection and care made every moment of my stay memorable in Wellington.

My greatest sources of strength are my parents. Ma motivated me to carry on when, at times, I was on the point of giving up. Baba remains my pillar.

My deepest gratitude goes to Abhik for allowing me to pursue research that often implied prolonged separation from him. His intellectual curiosity and love for the discipline of history inspired me deeply and sustained me intellectually in the bleakest of times.

# Abbreviations

| | |
|---|---|
| AIIHPH | All India Institute of Hygiene and Public Health |
| AIWC | All India Women's Conference |
| BHWC | Bengal Health Welfare Committee |
| CMC | Calcutta Medical College |
| GMC | General Medical Council |
| GOI | Government of India |
| IMS | Indian Medical Service |
| LMS | Licentiate in Medicine and Surgery |
| MB | Bachelor of Medicine |
| NAI | National Archives of India |
| SNDMA | Saroj Nalini Dutt Memorial Association |
| VLMS | Vernacular Licentiate in Medicine and Surgery |
| WBSA | West Bengal State Archives |
| WMS | Women's Medical Service |

# Introduction

It is sometimes argued that child-bearing is a normal physiological process of the body, automatic, self-regulating and entirely remote from disease. Ideally this may be so, but without the doctor and the nurse this process is associated with a maternal mortality in the neighbourhood of 25 per 1000, and an infantile mortality which in India may be as high as 35 per cent . . . Clearly if the medical profession are not to see obstetrics pass from their hands to the midwives, it is essential that they undertake to attend cases of childbirth, not only in those hospitals and maternity homes to which they have access, but also in the house of the people, and much of this work among the poorer classes must of necessity be free and subsidised.[1]

This statement by Major G. G. Jolly, the then director general of the Indian Medical Service (IMS)[2] in an address to the Delhi Maternity Services Co-ordination Committee in 1940, succinctly brings out the essence of medicalisation of childbirth. Medicalisation has been defined by a contemporary anthropologist Cecilia Van Hollen as 'the process whereby the medical establishment, as an institution with standardised professional guidelines, incorporates birth in the category of disease and requires that a medical professional oversees the birth process and determines treatment'.[3] It implies the rise of an interventionist approach to pregnancy as a pathological rather than a physiological state, the institutionalisation of the doctor–patient relationship and the growth of intra-professional issues in the process. However, what Major Jolly contemplated was an expanded midwifery service that would not solely be embedded in the rigours and institutional trappings of hospitals and maternity homes but extend itself to the 'house of the people . . . among the poorer classes', a social reconfiguration of obstetrics that in Jolly's vision would be integral to the assertion of professional control over pregnancy and childbirth. True to Jolly's vision, midwifery services in India had by the 1940s traversed into a new realm that worked towards a more effective management of birth through careful monitoring and a more holistic approach towards pregnant women's well-being. Such trends call for a reconsideration of existing historical narratives that pivoted around a narrow definition of medicalisation of childbirth in the colonial context.

Medicalisation of childbirth in the colonial context has so far been identified with three key themes: the attempt to reform or 'sanitise' the *zenana* (secluded quarters of a respectable household inhabited by its women) as the chief site of birthing practices, establishing lying-in *purdah* (literal meaning curtain, denoting seclusion) hospitals that were supervised by female doctors and, most significantly, replacing the allegedly 'barbaric' 'ignorant' traditional birth attendants or *dhais* with trained midwives and qualified female doctors.[4] Using Bengal as a case study, the book goes beyond this conventional narrative and traces the beginning of medicalisation of childbirth in the process of inclusion of midwifery as an academic subject at the Calcutta Medical College (CMC). It argues that the introduction of midwifery education at the Medical College reshaped existing views on birthing practice and went on to reflect a wider and more profound sociopolitical movement that eventually took shape at the behest of multiple actors operating mostly outside the orbit of colonial governance.

Feminist writings on midwifery and childbirth that burgeoned in the 1970s as a spin-off of the women's health movement in the West resent the marginalisation of midwives in the 'authoritative space' of 'hi-tech' births of the twentieth century. Such a space is allegedly controlled by the doctors and the hospital staff thereby curbing the autonomy of the midwife and the female patient.[5] Sheila Kitzinger speaking in favour of restoring the midwives to their traditional role asserted that the subordination of midwives to the doctors and the hospital administration has not only alienated women from the bodily and intimate experience of giving birth, but also led to the entire hospital administration being driven by the selfish concerns of 'financial stability, economy and functional efficiency'.[6] The consequence was, as she claimed, little reduction in the maternal mortality rates; in certain instances, maternal rates were lower in home-births supervised by midwives.[7] This book does not gauge the impact of medicalisation of pregnancy on the personal experiences of women in Bengal; such personal narratives are sparse and therefore hard to come by. The book does not also delve into the ethical question of whether professionalisation of midwifery alienated Bengali women from their bodily and emotional experience of giving birth under the 'comforting' presence of the midwife. It rather commits itself to analysing such factors that facilitated the transition of birth from a female-oriented ritual to a medical event. Thus the role of rhetoric, nationalist politics and certain institutions (such as the CMC and the Calcutta Municipal Corporation) in catapulting pregnancy and childbirth to the centre of nation-building endeavours assumes centrality in the analyses.

A key aim of the book is to analyse how medicalisation of childbirth was intrinsically shaped by the social reform movement of the nineteenth century and nationalist politics and colonial public health policies of the twentieth century. At the same time, it seeks to decentre itself from Christian missionaries as the prime agents of modernisation of birthing practices, especially in the early years of colonial rule, and locate midwifery training and practices within a wider and more complex range of social drivers.[8] In the twentieth century, as the book argues, the profession of obstetrics came to constitute an ever-expanding space mediated by a wide range of actors such as the medical professionals, middle-class women activists and the local self-governing bodies who were influenced as much by nationalism and colonial public health policies as by global discourses on health. In analysing the shifting strands of midwifery practice in Bengal over a period of eighty years, the study seeks to discern the process through which Bengali women's body that was once perceived as the citadel of physical modesty and cultural purity and, hence, shielded from public sight by patriarchal norms of seclusion, became by the end of colonial period, a subject of intense medical, public and nationalist scrutiny.

The notion that Bengal's rendezvous with the West shaped the contours of its early colonial intellectual history has remained deeply embedded in existing historical writings. The reigning tendency, for a long time, has been to trace the beginning of Bengal's tryst with modernity to a creative phase of intellectual awakening and linguistic and literary modernisation that is referred to as the Renaissance.[9] However, recent researches have challenged the linear trajectory of Bengal's cultural transformation and literary modernisation by arguing how the spawning of an entire corpus of cheap vernacular literature within the same time frame paved the way for more variegated forms of literary and cultural expressions that seldom fitted into the parameters set by modern renaissance literature.[10] The cognisance of the pluralistic nature of Bengal's cultural transformations has now led to the agency and autonomy of the 'local' being acknowledged in unequivocal terms.

Notwithstanding the persistence of the indigenous and the local as dominant social forces in colonial times, the hegemonic influence of western scientific thought in redefining existing sociocultural categories and in allowing new structures of knowledge to emerge can hardly be glossed over. The colossal impact of 'scientific' consciousness and rationalisation of thought in nineteenth-century Bengal is illustrative of this fact. Scientific impulse of the newly colonised middle-class Bengalis was central to triggering momentous socio-economic transformations as well as in initiating more enduring processes of the re-ordering of the society along certain 'modern' parameters. What the book attempts to demonstrate is how the access of the newly colonised middle class or the *bhadralok* (literal meaning gentleman) to certain contraptions of colonial modernity such as English education, colonial professional world and, most significantly, the print culture turned out to be powerful stimulants in investing them with a 'rational' consciousness and imbuing certain dormant social issues with a sense of urgency and transparency that had not existed in the pre-colonial era.

It is also argued that the transplantation of western science onto the colony did not represent a linear route resulting in the marginalisation or complete erasure of the pre-existing indigenous/local knowledge. It rather embodied a mutually constitutive dialogue between the western and the local by which new and sometimes 'hybridised' forms of knowledge were generated.[11] By the same token the infiltration of western medical knowledge into existing local medical traditions entailed a dynamic interpenetration of two distinct systems of thoughts that caused both of them to lose some of their steadfastness and undergo a continuous process of reformulation and re-articulation in a bid to complement or replace each other.[12] The unravelling of an entire gamut of vernacular 'medical' literature demonstrates a vibrant co-mingling of the western and the local.[13] It is not the intention of the book to analyse how birth became a site of rigorous contestation in competing medical discourses in Bengal. This book rather seeks to understand the extent to which western medical paradigm, despite its co-existence with competing medical traditions, guided the transition of midwifery from a cultural phenomena in the nineteenth century to an overtly westernised and professionalised science of obstetrics in the twentieth century.

In the early nineteenth century, Bengal's well-entrenched medical establishment along the lines of western scientific medicine could boast of being ahead of both Madras and Bombay Presidencies. The foundation of the CMC in 1835 was, according to Mel Gorman, a shining proof of Bengal's transforming social conditions and receptivity to western ideas and practices.[14] Yet Bengal lagged behind Madras in the sphere of midwifery education. Madras was far ahead of Bengal and Bombay in terms of the popularity of its state-sponsored lying-in hospital which was established in 1844. The Madras hospital prided itself on creating a class of trained Indian midwives who practised successfully in various parts of the Madras Presidency. The superior quality of the Madras Lying-In Hospital, according to Sean Lang, 'proved a useful weapon for the Government of Madras in its long-running rivalry with the presidencies of Bombay and especially Bengal'.[15] In Bengal, on the contrary, a lying-in ward was established in 1841 but its success in training the dhais was rather dubious. The training of dhais was again instituted in the Dacca Mitford Hospital in the 1870s, being greeted with much optimism.[16] Piecemeal efforts were also made by the CMC from the 1860s to the 1870s and by the Eden Hospital in the 1880s, but such endeavours were never as successful in Bengal as in Madras and later in Punjab, Sindh and a few other states.[17]

Bengal's tardy response to reforming midwifery was perceived as a consequence of the long-standing Bengali perception of childbirth and women's health as exclusively 'female-regulated domains' that were guarded by practice of seclusion (purdah) and, therefore, impenetrable by western medicine.[18] Similar perceptions prevailed in nineteenth-century Europe where midwifery was 'stigmatised' as part of women's everyday domestic and reproductive functions.[19] However, in Bengal, purdah was a more convenient trope frequently resorted to by the government and the CMC authorities in justifying their reluctance to finance the institutionalisation of midwifery. The colonial government was apparently more intent on safeguarding the health of the army and the European population than tending to the physical well-being of native women.[20] How much of the process of institutionalisation of midwifery was hindered by the presumed cultural constraints in the Bengali society? Who generated the debate to reform midwifery and transform it into the specialised science of obstetrics? In answering the questions the book explores three discursive strands that explain the constitution of a medical discourse on pregnancy and childbirth and also the factors that underscored the institutionalisation and professionalisation of midwifery in Bengal in the twentieth century.

## A new middle-class discourse on midwifery in the popular print

The impulse for modernising childbirth in nineteenth-century Bengal stemmed from an embattled response of a new colonised and increasingly self-conscious middle class that was, time and again, disconcerted by the colonial critique of Bengali society and customs. The Brahmos, a reformist group of liberal disposition, redirected their reformist initiatives towards dismantling the colonial conviction that any society that undervalued women was decidedly inferior in the hierarchy of civilisations.[21] The impetus for reform also emanated from certain 'indigenous reasons'. The customs of *sati*, ban on widow remarriage and *kulin* polygamy that often resulted in child widowhood led to a large number of women being left barren and were, therefore, held responsible by reformers, some of whom belonged to *kulin* Brahmin families, for the dwindling number of *kulins*.[22] Women being denied the agency to articulate themselves in the first half of the nineteenth century, the early polemics on women's status were confined to a constricted realm of male patriarchal engagement with colonial modernity.[23]

Women's health and childbearing being perceived as quotidian aspects of female-centred domesticity did not figure in the reformist agenda of the first half of the nineteenth century. Yet childbirth did evolve as a 'visible' area of concern in Bengal in the second half of the century, thanks to the emergence of a public sphere that was nurtured and sustained by the growth of a vibrant print culture from the 1860s. Commenting on the importance of the print culture in shaping middle-class identity, Tanika Sarkar states that,

> Print revolutionised reading habits and possibilities . . . within the confines of a limited class, reading became a non-specialised, fluid, pervasive, everyday activity . . . a cross-section of thinking men, and even a few exceptionally fortunate women, could, without formal learning, develop and express ideas within a public debate over the shape of their own daily lives.[24]

Print brought into the public sphere issues such as marriage, domesticity and childbearing practices that were previously relegated to the sequestered realms of the private sphere. The publication of an increasing number of vernacular literary and women's magazines enabled the forging of an autonomous space for the Bengali intelligentsia within which cultural and social issues, including the latent ones, were debated and imbued with a degree of criticality that had not existed before. Despite being tainted by nationalist sentiments, such debates seldom impinged on direct political activity.[25]

The new socio-economic conditions of existence ushered in by colonial rule prompted reconfiguration of the role of women as 'helpmates' and enlightened companions.[26] The Census of 1872 testified to a growing number of Bengali males moving out of their native districts to Calcutta and its neighbourhoods in search of clerical jobs in 'commercial houses' and 'public offices'.[27] For many such middle-class professionals, repositioning of women as enlightened wives and mothers in a reformed domestic terrain became integral to the process of adjustment to the altered conditions of existence under colonial regime.

Victorian ideas of domesticity profoundly influenced the restructuring of domesticity, familial relations and the hygienic and health practices in the Bengali household. Reason became central to the process of reforming domesticity and reconceptualising a new enlightened woman (who came to be known as *bhadramahila*) as opposed to the traditional women of the past. Motherhood was integral to the definition of the new woman or bhadramahila. Writings on maternity and childcare such as Shib Chunder Deb's *Sisu Palan* ('Child Rearing') or Gangaprasad Mukhopadhyay's *Matrishiksha* ('Education of Mother') were in wide circulation from the 1860s.[28] As early as 1867, *Bamabodhini Patrika*, the earliest women's magazine run by the Brahmos, denounced the practice of choosing the 'smallest' and the most 'ill-ventilated' room as the site of birth (*anturghar*) which, according to it, was the sign of 'irrational' practices of the 'uneducated' women causing the death of newborn infants.[29]

Parallel to the creation of a professional middle class and their access to western education and colonial professional sphere was the emergence of a new medical culture that was fostered by the foundation of the CMC. The new medical culture provided the middle class with a coherent discursive framework within which existing health practices were interrogated and new knowledge practices were accepted and conceded greater space. The new knowledge practices essentially centred on the introduction of medical instruments like thermometer and stethoscope and on the initiation of new discursive modes such as hospital training, clinical-anatomy and maintaining case records. The novel elements thus introduced into the medical curriculum came to constitute the core of 'hospital medicine'.[30] The introduction of anatomic dissection, in particular, ushered in profound epistemic transformations in the perception of body and disease. In the long run, clinical-anatomy became the principal driving force behind the emergence of a new medical culture in India that based itself on a wide array of medical and surgical practices and paved the way for the institutionalisation and 'hierarchisation' of doctor–patient relationship, in a manner quite unknown in the pre-colonial era.

In the initial years following the foundation of the CMC, the graduates and the faculties of the College rejoiced over anatomy as the most clinching evidence of the superiority of western medicine over existing medical practices. Commenting on the success of candidates at the Medical College in scoring high marks in the newly introduced subjects of anatomy and physiology, Professor Goodeve Chuckerburty proudly stated, with particular reference to practical anatomy:

> That the prejudices of ages should, in six short months, have been overthrown, and the iron bonds of a most debasing and mischievous superstition have been thus suddenly burst asunder by a few simple youths, aided only by the force of a superior education, was, indeed, a spectacle worthy to behold. . . . We felt that the great obstacle to the advancement of the institution under our charge was surmounted, and that the objects for which the College was established were even now fulfilled.[31]

In the next few decades, anatomy established itself as the linchpin of western medical discourse underscoring major epistemic shifts in knowledge practices. It had far-reaching implications for the society at large, redefining the parameters of health practices in Bengal. It induced middle-class interest in the mechanisms of body that became abundantly manifest in the profusion of writings and diagrammatic expressions of human body that began to inundate popular print from the 1860s.

Knowing the body constituted an integral part of female education through home tutoring. Essays on biological functions of human body and rational redefinition of health practices were in circulation in the women's magazines from the second half of the nineteenth century. From 1867 onwards, such writings called for the uprooting of midwifery from the complex field of rituals and cultural practices and redefined it as a medical science. In the context of England, Ornella Moscucci's *The Science of Woman: Gynaecology and Gender in England, 1800–1929* explicates how the medical profession gradually assumed control over the domain of childbirth and women's diseases by citing the scientific nature of its claims about women's physiology as being inherently pathological.[32] Such trends were visible in Bengal where the medical profession clamoured for medicalisation of childbirth by disseminating medical–scientific knowledge about pregnancy and childbirth through the popular women's magazines and health journals and projecting such knowledge as superior to the existing female-oriented knowledge practices surrounding childbirth.

Bengali women's magazines such as *Bamabodhini Patrika, Antahpur, Bangamahila* and *Bharati*[33] offer meaningful insights into the identity imaginings of the colonised elites and their complex negotiations with modernity beyond the key sites of colonial power. Being usually composed by Bengali male reformers, the articles in such magazines highlighted male perceptions of the redefined role of women as enlightened wives and mothers under the new patriarchy. Gradually, women's health was perceived as central to the ordering of the emerging idea of nation and the nationalist reconfiguration of family. Female body constituted a fertile site on which the disciplining of the private sphere (as represented by the family) and the public sphere (as epitomised by incipient ideas of an emerging nation) was negotiated. Towards the end of the nineteenth century the perceptions of literate women on health, maternity and childbirth were beginning to be documented as veritable part of the process by which female subjectivity was constituted.

While the foundation of the CMC and attempts at reforming midwifery indicate unimpeded flow of western medical ideas into the sociocultural fabric of Bengali life, the consolidation of conservative forces in the 1870s confounded this process. The assertion of a distinctly Hindu identity from the 1870s and the selected revival of some of the traditional practices of the past whipped up a powerful anti-colonial backlash that stood to repudiate all that were overtly associated with the West.[34] The unleashing of the conservative forces emboldened male patriarchal control over Hindu wives whose bodies were imagined as pure and unscathed by colonialism.[35] In this particular milieu, western allopathic medicine[36] identified as state medicine jostled for space in popular print along with other medical discourses such as Ayurveda and Homeopathy. As allopathy was being censured as a colonial import, women were consciously portrayed as repositories of indigenous medical knowledge. Drawing upon the prevailing cultural revivalist mood of the time, a certain section of the bhadralok sought to protect the 'uncolonised' domestic terrain from colonial intervention that accounted for the fervent opposition of the Bengalis to raising the age of marriage of girls from ten to twelve years. The resultant Age of Consent Controversy of 1890 is all too well traversed in existing historiography to be elaborated here. Suffice it to mention that while at the peak of the controversy, the revivalist-nationalists slighted medical opinion on the evils of child marriage and early maternity and prioritised *Shastric* injunctions on the need for retaining the purity of female body; debates on child marriage and early maternity continued to surface in the nationalist discourse of the early twentieth century and crucially shaped public perception of maternal and infant health in Bengal.

One of the objectives of the book is to analyse the extent to which literate Bengali women internalised the male discourse on modernity with regards to issues such as the ills surrounding childbirth, child marriage and early maternity. The presumption that the debates on the condition of women ceased to figure in the nationalist agenda in the second half of the nineteenth century due to the 'nationalist resolution of the women's question' had maintained its undisputed sway in historical imaginations for a fairly long time.[37] Partha Chatterjee, the most forceful exponent of this view, deemed it as nationalism's success in situating the 'women's question' in an 'inner domain of sovereignty, far removed from the arena of political contest with the colonial state'.[38] In recent years, this uncritical assumption of women's silent acquiescence to the nationalist resolution of women's question has been challenged by scholars. Himani Bannerji, for instance, has argued that women far from complying with their newly assigned role as the upholder of the sanctuary of home were in reality drawn more towards reason, education and politics.[39] Equally strong was their propensity to flout the norms of patriarchy, a fact repeatedly drawn to attention by other researches that highlight the various subversive ways in which women sought to critique the social inequalities experienced by them.[40] Drawing upon Bannerji's argument, the study seeks to answer the following questions: Did the response of the bhadramahila signify a tacit approbation of the male reformist discourse? To what extent did they voice critiques of male-approved social customs? How did the Indian middle-class women in the 1920s and 1930s respond to the nationalist discourse on scientific management of birth and the medical profession's promotion of the idea of medical supervision of pregnancy?

## Institutionalising midwifery

The transition of midwifery from a lay art into a specialised branch of medical science underscores major epistemological shifts that could only be effected through incorporation of midwifery into the formal educational structure. One of the cardinal aims of the book is to analyse the various axes along which midwifery was recast into a medical discipline and subsequently institutionalised and sustained in Bengal. The proceedings of the Medical and Education branch under the General, Municipal, Judicial and Local Self-Government Department of the Government of Bengal from the 1860s to 1940s reveal the fervent debates amongst colonial medical officials surrounding midwifery education in the nineteenth century and, in the process, sheds light on the nature of colonial governance in India and the priorities that guided the British officials in the various phases of colonial rule.

Financial considerations, the book will progressively demonstrate, were a clinching factor in the formulation of policies towards health, education and other such tertiary areas.

A predominant tendency in existing historical scholarship on medicalisation of childbirth in India is to offer a gendered narrative that presupposes the absence of male physicians' involvement in childbirth as a condition generated by the peculiar cultural custom of seclusion. The deeply entrenched practice of seclusion, it is argued, prevented female patients from seeking medical care from men. It has become almost perfunctory to assume that the impenetrability of the zenana led to female medical education being prioritised in India and facilitated the trend towards professionalisation of women doctors in Britain. Antoinette Burton, for instance, has argued that the long held belief of Indian women trapped in 'unhygienic Oriental Zenana' proved to be the central motivating factor in the 'institutionalisation of women's medicine and the professionalisation of women doctors in Victorian Britain'. The British medical women waged a dual battle against male dominance in institutionalised medicine in Britain and against the less-qualified women medical missionaries. For these women doctors trained in the London School of Medicine for Women, providing medical care to Indian women 'imprisoned' in Zenana and projecting it as an imperial obligation was the only viable way to salvage their professional career.[41]

The colonial scheme to train indigenous women in Bengal as midwives, doctors and hospital assistants is perceived as an imperial attempt 'to penetrate the zenana, not with force but with the forceps of the lady doctors'.[42] Therefore the assertion that 'Due to the stricter separation of sexes in Bengal than in the west, male dominated medical science was less involved in improving the conditions of mothers and babies, upper-middle class families apart' has dominated existing scholarship on the subject.[43] Chandrika Paul's historical study of Bengali women in the medical profession in the nineteenth century and Supriya Guha's latest research on the subject further reinforce the contention that the female doctors in Bengal were the sole mediators between the *antahpur* (inner secluded parts of the house) and the outside world.[44]

To assume that female doctors were the only conduit through which western medical ideas penetrated Bengali middle-class homes is rather preposterous, given the indisputable fact that new scientific ideas of midwifery were diffused into the inner sanctums of Bengali homes through the popular print, which was for a long period of time controlled by enlightened males. Striving to offer a more nuanced perspective, the study contends that gender differentials were not integral to understanding the transition in midwifery education and practices that took place in the nineteenth and twentieth centuries, and that a more balanced understanding of the role of both male and female doctors in medicalising childbirth is both plausible and desirable. Of late, revisionist historians have called for a fine-tuning of approach towards the history of women's health care arguing that the very tendency to gender obstetric practices is a cultural phenomenon and that there is nothing biological about women seeking treatment from a member of their own sex.[45] This study seeks to implant itself in such broader historical currents. It aims to position the female and male medical professionals in their respective spheres of dominance. While the preponderance of female doctors in obstetrics and gynaecology is extolled as a sign of the absence of 'masculinisation' of obstetrics in India, the moot question that eludes existing historiography is: Did the female doctors deviate much from the ethos guiding the male-controlled medical set-up in the West? The answer is in the negative. The female doctors undeniably gained easier access to the Indian zenanas and might have won the confidence of middle- and upper-class women with much more ease than male doctors but in preaching the gospel of scientific birth they echoed the opinion and priorities of male medical establishment.

The book delves into the critical task of exploring the multifarious ways in which male doctors sustained themselves in the profession by defining the parameters of scientific midwifery. Despite their presence in the profession of obstetrics being less justified on cultural grounds than their female counterparts, the huge volume of writings left behind by them reveal their agency in spreading western medical ideas in Bengali households and in educating dhais in consonance with western knowledge practices. It is interesting to note how, for instance, professional medical journals published in the Bengali language such as *Bishak Darpan* and *Cikitsa Prakasa* offered a platform for the more localised male general practitioners to acquire knowledge about midwifery in the light of received ideas from the West and apply them to local conditions.

## Professionalising midwifery in the interwar years

The study delineates the contours of professionalisation of midwifery in the twentieth century and the specific historical context conditioning it. Attempts to formulate a single cogent definition of the term 'profession' have persistently baffled sociologists who continue to wrestle with the theoretical formulations of the term and the various meanings conveyed by it. Eliot Friedson while acknowledging the lack of consensus amongst sociologists has arrived at a more balanced definition. Friedson defines profession as 'an agent of formal knowledge', one that can be distinguished from other occupations by virtue of its formal knowledge which it applies, develops and protects.[46] He further cautions us of the need to use the term 'profession' in a specific 'historical and national sense'.[47]

Drawing insights from Friedson's definition, the book aims to explore the sociopolitical context in which midwifery was professionalised in Bengal. It seeks to understand whether or not the drive to professionalise midwifery emanated from the broader and globally relevant eugenic ideas of 'racial regeneration' and 'national welfare' that came to inform nationalist debates on public health in India in the interwar years. The *Swadeshi* movement that was launched in 1907 as a mark of protest against the partition of Bengal in 1905 by Lord Curzon brought to the foreground the nationalist imagination of Bengal and later India.[48] The rhetoric of nation-as-mother gained currency in the aftermath of this movement. In this milieu, maternal and infant mortality acquired centre stage in the nationalist discourse since loss of maternal and infant life challenged Bengal's and then India's viability as a nation.

The ideologies of nationhood were transmitted through the new rhetoric of nationalism that was directly connected with Bengali middle-class aspirations for power and hegemony. Yet nationalist thought could not be considered as independent of post-Enlightenment bourgeois-rationalist knowledge, which wove a web of colonial domination in the garb of universalism.[49] The book argues that despite promoting medicalisation of childbirth in nationalist terms, the movement for maternal and infant welfare that was spearheaded by Bengali medical professionals and public health workers in the interwar years embraced a rational approach towards birth that drew heavily on western medical science and technology and, hence, remained firmly ensconced in the post-Enlightenment bourgeois-rationalist approach. Concerns for nation and future of the race were frequently voiced in the vernacular magazines from the beginning of the twentieth century and became an emotive subject when linked to the imagery of nation-as-mother. The census reports, the annual reports of the Health Officer of the Calcutta Municipal Corporation and the reports of the Public Health Commissioner of Bengal revealed high infant mortality rates in Bengal adding to the fear of the nationalists. The study attempts to understand how the issue of infant and maternal mortality that acquired centrality in the Bengali public discourse of nationalism was linked to the questions of reforming birthing practices and professionalising midwifery in the interwar years.

By examining popular health magazines such as *Svasthya Samacara*, *Svasthya* and *Cikitsa Sammilani* that regularly discussed the myriad challenges posed by maternal and infant mortality through the prism of nationalism and eugenics, the book analyses the extent to which the debates initiated by practitioners of western medicine reflected the extent of the internalisation of western medical discourse by the colonised elites.[50] As the subscription lists of such journals and magazines indicate, such magazines pandered largely to a non-medical lay public including eminent zamindars, lawyers and teachers.

The intersection of the national and the global is central to understanding the trend towards professionalisation of midwifery in the interwar years. Articles from popular health magazine like *Svasthya Samacara* were replete with examples from far-off countries like America, New Zealand and Europe suggesting that the modernity the middle-class Bhadralok were trying to embrace emanated not only from close association with the British colonial rulers but also from a global awareness of similar transitions experienced by various other countries in the late nineteenth and early twentieth centuries.

In the post-1918 years, maternal and child health assumed greater significance in the Bengali public discourse, reflecting similar concerns in England about the dwindling physical strength of the soldiers that sparked off initiatives to save infant life. Interests in preserving infant life had long been expressed in England with the improvement in the standard of public health work, more prominently since the Anglo-South African (Boer) War of 1899. In the post-1918 years, the value of maternal life as a factor determining the birth of healthy infants was increasingly realised and brought to the fore. It became entwined with eugenic discourse on the improvement of race. To what extent did the concerns for maternal life in Bengal reflect global eugenic discourse of the time that argued about the centrality of race in the process of national regeneration? What was the specific nature of the argument on racial improvement that took shape in Bengali nationalist discourse? How were the nationalist rhetoric of motherhood and race deployed by the Bengali doctors in the interwar years in promoting professionalisation of obstetrics? The study focuses, in particular, on the role of medical professionals, both male and female, in linking the demands for professionalisation of midwifery to the broader social reform movements and nationalist politics that also significantly concerned the condition of women in society and public health issues in Bengal in the interwar years.

In England, as Jane Lewis has argued, the national concerns for maternal and child welfare work were duly seized by obstetricians in promoting medicalised childbirth and, in the process, advancing their own 'neglected speciality'.[51] The threat posed by maternal and infant mortality was perceived solely in terms of maternity statistics, and seen as 'discrete medical problems' to be solved through the provision of health visitors, improved maternity services and infant welfare centres. In the process, the social, environmental and economic causes underlying the higher mortality rates were overlooked.[52] Such trends were evident in Bengal. While the nationalists blamed the economic policies of the government for the higher mortality rates, the government denounced the social customs of the Bengalis. The obstetricians, however, blamed both and sought the remedy in medicalisation of childbirth and improved maternity services. The study will examine how the intense nationalist politics in Bengal in the interwar years shaped the public health discourse on maternal and child welfare from the perspective of the indigenous medical profession in Bengal. The English language medical journals such as the *Indian Medical Gazette* which was the mouthpiece of colonial medical establishment[53] and also private journals edited independently by Indian doctors such as the *Calcutta Medical Journal, the Journal of the Indian Medical Association* and *the Indian Medical Record* are integral to understanding the perceptions of Bengali medical professionals and the idioms deployed by them in promoting medical control over birth. Similarly, the *Journal of the Association for Medical Women in India* represents the views of medical women in India on a wide variety of issues ranging from maternal and infant health to gender-based professional issues.

Did this emerging discourse on maternal and infant health facilitate the trend towards technological intervention in women's reproductive health in Bengal? Were the concepts of 'reformed woman' and 'healthy mother', popularised by social reformers and politicians, also becoming the discursive terrains where the Bengali bhadralok and the medical establishment were strengthening their patriarchal and professional control, respectively? In answering these questions, the study brings to light the pivotal role of the Calcutta Municipal Corporation and the Public Health Department in professionalising midwifery in the interwar years. By instituting domiciliary midwifery services and establishing a chain of maternity homes that sought to provide professional medical care for pregnant women across class and religious divides, the Corporation contributed towards the creation of a professional structure that was premised on the institutionalisation of western scientific medicine. Even the midwives who were trained under the auspices of the Corporation for domiciliary maternity services were integrated into this professional framework and became the dispensers of western knowledge which had, by then, acquired the status of 'formal knowledge'.

The institutional expansion and professionalisation of western-style midwifery in India has so far been unanimously identified with the foundation in 1885 of the 'National Association for Supplying Female Medical Aid to the Women of India', better known as the Dufferin Fund. Founded by Lady Dufferin, the wife of the Viceroy, the Fund was conceived as a training programme under official patronage with the explicit aim of providing medical training to nurses and midwives and extending medical relief through dispensaries, female wards, female doctors and female hospitals. The Fund has been labelled as the single most important step in the institutionalisation of medicine for women in India.[54]

The book argues that the history of institutionalisation of midwifery is not solely the story of Dufferin Fund whose very operation was deeply splintered along class lines. While the exclusivist approach of the Fund served to curb the colonising potential of western medicine, there were other channels through which western medicine infiltrated Indian homes by cutting across class and religious divides. In illustrating this point, the book examines closely the role of the Calcutta Municipal Corporation. It derives major theoretical insights from W. R. Arney's powerful sociological analysis on the forming of the profession of obstetrics. Arney has noted how the profession of obstetrics experienced significant conceptual shifts in the wake of the Second World War in terms of managing pregnancy. It began to prioritise surveillance and monitoring over birth. During this phase, obstetrics moved out of hospitals and extended into larger geographical spaces so that 'all the events in a woman's life up to the point of birth became obstetrical data; all the events after birth became potential material worthy of study and incorporation into the obstetrical project'.[55]

The Calcutta Municipal Corporation and its manifold activities pertaining to midwifery services decentred obstetrics from hospitals and maternity homes by introducing a wide array of novel practices such as home-visits and domiciliary midwifery services that drew lower-middle-class women in Calcutta into the fold of professional medical care and the institutions promoting it such as maternity homes and welfare centres. As a result of these experiments, the scope of obstetrics expanded over larger geographical and social spaces even as slums and the lower-middle-class enclaves became the new sites of obstetric research on maternal morbidity and mortality in the interwar years and thereafter. Unlike the Dufferin Fund that has been dubbed as an 'intensely political organisation' with the purported motive to change Indian attitudes towards western medicine and British rule, the maternity schemes of the Calcutta Municipal Corporation were conceived and implemented by indigenous elites.[56]

Concerns over maternal and infant mortality led to antenatal care being prioritised by the medical professionals in the interwar years, although such ideas were sporadically in circulation in the popular magazines in the nineteenth century. In laying the groundwork for antenatal care, Bengal drew upon English examples. The evolution of antenatal care in post-Industrial Revolution England, as Ann Oakley has demonstrated, was part of the broader preoccupation of the state with questions of 'public health' and 'national welfare'. Oakley shows how, in collusion with the state, which took care of the social and economic reorganisation of medical work, the medical profession strategically deployed technology as a weapon to fortify its professional claims over women's bodies and choices with regard to childbirth. The central message that emerged was 'that pregnant women were themselves deficient: they lacked the necessary intelligence, foresight, education or responsibility to see that the only proper pathway to successful motherhood was the one repeatedly surveyed by medical expertise'.[57] The book will analyse the extent to which the trope of maternal ignorance was deployed in asserting patriarchal and professional control over women's bodies in Bengal. Yet unlike Oakley's study which confined itself to analysing the impact of invasive medical procedures on women mostly belonging to the affluent class, antenatal care in Bengal in the period under review was less about applying invasive medical technology and more about providing cheaper and yet more effective alternative to doctor-supervised hospital birth.

## Roadmap

The chapters are arranged thematically. The first chapter looks at the social–intellectual environment within which an indigenous scientific discourse on birthing practices and midwifery was constructed in Bengal between the 1860s and 1900. It analyses the contribution of the popular Bengali print media in extending western medical ideas into the culturally secluded sections of Bengali homes. Drawing upon a wide range of popular magazines, the chapter outlines the preoccupation of the Bengali middle class with health and the colonial stigma of effeminacy that haunted the middle class throughout the nineteenth century. Concerns for infant mortality and the need to ensure the birth of healthy babies were seen as a corrective to the sense of degeneracy haunting the Bengali bhadralok. Consequently, birthing practices, along with other broader issues of domesticity, conjugality and reconceptualisation of women, were brought to the centre of a vigorous public debate. The chapter also captures the responses of some educated women towards such social debates concerning their health conditions.

The second chapter examines the processes through which midwifery was institutionalised and evolved into a medical discipline and an academic subject in Bengal between the 1860s and the 1930s. The various axes around which midwifery was institutionalised included the colonial scheme to train the dhais at the CMC and Eden Hospital. It was followed by the steps taken since 1882 by the College authorities to introduce medical education to women. The chapter brings to light the agency of male doctors in strengthening the discipline of obstetrics through research, experimentation with modern surgical techniques and disseminating such ideas through tracts meant for popular reading and through monographs and essays published in medical journals for medical students. It also touches upon the rise of nationalist sentiments amongst the male doctors that became visible in the wake of the General Medical Council of London's decision to withdraw recognition of medical degrees of the Indian medical colleges in 1924.

The third chapter analyses the professionalisation of obstetrics in Bengal between 1900 and the 1940s. It begins by analysing the arguments of Bengali medical men whose concerns for infant mortality echoed eugenic ideas of racial degeneration. The solution was sought in medicalisation of childbirth and expansion of modern and professionalised midwifery services. The medical professionals were also at this stage actively seeking to extend their sphere of control over pregnant women's bodies in order to protect them from diseases during pregnancy and giving birth to 'weaklings'. The chapter discusses at length the role played by the Calcutta Municipal Corporation in laying the groundwork for modern maternity care accessible to females of all classes. It goes on to show how the sphere of professionalised obstetrics was shared by male and female doctors bound by common professional ethos.

The fourth chapter examines the growth of the idea of antenatal care in Bengal, roughly from 1900 till the 1940s. Rudimentary notions of antenatal care that were disseminated in women's magazines in the late nineteenth century came to be delivered in medical terms by the medical professionals in the interwar years. The chapter closely examines such writings on antenatal care in the popular women's magazines and health journals in the early twentieth century. The second part of it analyses the antenatal work done in Bengal which, lacking state support, was carried out through the initiatives of the Calcutta Municipal Corporation on a pattern similar to that of England and through voluntary bodies such as the Bengal branch of the Indian Red Cross Society, indicating the marginal nature of hospital-based antenatal care. In the ultimate analysis, due to paucity of sources, and despite a powerful public modernist discourse, antenatal care as it was provided to pregnant women in colonial Bengal was more about advice on diet, clothing and hygiene and less about actual facilities for doctor-supervised birth.

## Notes

1 G.G. Jolly, 'The Need for Co-operation in the Medical Health Services of India with Special Reference to Maternity and Child Welfare', *Indian Medical Gazette*, Vol. 75, No.236, April 1940, 236.
2 Major General G.G. Jolly was the director general of the IMS from 1939 to 1943 and became the chief commissioner of the Indian Red Cross Society. He was involved in the public health movement in India. His views were quoted by eminent nationalist obstetricians like Subodh Mitra in arguing for medical supervision of childbirth. Jolly's view was widely shared by the Bengali doctors in the 1930s and 1940s.
3 Cecilia Van Hollen, *Birth on the Threshold: Childhood and Modernity in South India*, New Delhi: Zubaan, 2003, 203.
4 Sarah Hodges, *Reproductive Health in India: History, Politics, Controversies*, Delhi: Orient Longman, 2006, 5.
5 See for example, Jean Donnison, *Midwives and Medical Men: A History of the Struggle for the Control of Childbirth*, Second Edition, London: Historical Publications Ltd, 1988. Published for the first time in 1977 and written largely from a feminist perspective, Jean Donnison's historical work traces the history of the institution of midwifery since ancient times and its gradual decline from the eighteenth century with the rise of forceps and male-midwifery. She resents the marginalisation of midwives in the authoritative space of 'high tech' births manoeuvred by obstetricians, anaesthetists and paediatrics; Jane B.Donnegan, *Women and Men Midwives: Medicine, Morality and Misogyny in Early America*, New York: Greenwood, 1978; Lianne McTavish, *Childbirth and the Display of Authority in Early Modern France*, Aldershot: Ashgate, 2005; Charlotte G. Borst, *Catching Babies: The Professionalisation of Childbirth, 1870–1920*, Cambridge, MA: Harvard University Press, 1996.
6 Sheila Kitzinger, *The Midwife Challenge*, Second Edition, London: Pandora Press, 1991.
7 Ibid.

8  The role of the female medical missionaries has been discussed in some of the following works: David Arnold, *Science, Technology and Medicine in Colonial India*, Cambridge: Cambridge University Press, 2000; Maina Chawla Singh, *Gender, Religion and 'Heathen Lands': American Missionary Women in South Asia (1860–1940s)*, New York: Garland, 2000; and recently Team Allender, *Learning Femininity in Colonial India, 1820–1932*, Manchester: Manchester University Press, 2000. Most of the medical missionary activities, as these books show, were based in North India and some part of the South, and *not* in Bengal per se.

9  The orientalists, as David Kopf describes, were a 'group of "acculturated" civil, military and judicial officials (and some missionaries)' who worked as the representatives of the British nation in the early history of the establishment of colonial rule in India, that is roughly between the 1770s and the 1830s. The Orientalists were not concerned with preserving exclusive racial privilege and distance from the natives. Hence, they formed 'enduring relations' with the 'Bengali intelligentsia to whom they served as sources for knowledge of the West and with whom they worked to promote social and cultural change in Calcutta'. See David Kopf, *British Orientalism and the Bengal Renaissance*, Berkeley and Los Angeles: University of California Press, 1969, 3–5.

10  Anindita Ghosh, 'Revisiting the "Bengal Renaissance": Literary Bengali and Low-Life Print in Colonial Calcutta', *Economic and Political Weekly*, Vol.37, No.2, 2002, 19–25.

11  Kapil Raj, *Relocating Modern Science: Circulation and the Construction of Knowledge in South Asia and Europe, 1650–1900*, Houndmills and New York: Palgrave Macmillan, 2007; Pradip Kumar Bose, ed. *Health and Society in Bengal: A Selection from Late 19th-Century Bengali Periodicals*, New Delhi: Sage, 2006.

12  Bose, *Health and Society in Bengal*, see Introduction.

13  Projit Bihari Mukharji, *Nationalising the Body: Medical Market, Print and Daktari Medicine*, London: Anthem Press, 2011.

14  Mel Gorman, 'Introduction of Western Science into Colonial India: Role of the CMC', *Proceedings of the American Philosophical Society*, Vol.128, No.2, 1988, 276–298.

15  Sean Lang, 'Drop the Demon Dai: Maternal Mortality and the State in Colonial Madras, 1840–1875', *Social History of Medicine*, Vol.18, No.3, 2005, 377.

16  Editorial, 'Dhatribidyalayer Biboron', *Bamabodhini Patrika*, Vol.6, No.89, December 1871, 269–270.

17  The earliest effort to train the dhais began in Amritsar in 1866 with the establishment of the Amritsar Dhai's School which was under the Church of English Zenana Missionary Society. Geraldine Forbes, 'Education to Earn: Training Women in the Medical Professions', in Geraldine Forbes, ed. *Women in Colonial India: Essays on Politics, Medicine, and Historiography*, New Delhi: Chronicle Books, 2005, 106–107.

18  Margaret Ida Balfour and Ruth Young, *The Work of Medical Women in India*, Oxford: Oxford University Press, 1929, WBSA (West Bengal State Archives), Proceedings of the Lieutenant Governor of Bengal, General Department, Medical Branch, Progs Nos.1–7, August 1867.

19 Ann Oakley, 'Wise woman and Medicine Man: Changes in the Management of Childbirth', in Juliet Mitchell and Ann Oakley, eds. *The Rights and Wrongs of Women*, Middlesex: Penguin Books, 1976, 33.

20 David Arnold, *Colonising the Body: State Medicine and Epidemic Disease in Nineteenth-Century India*, Berkeley, Los Angeles and London: University of California Press, 1993.

21 James Mill was one of the chief exponents of this view. He famously stated, 'Among rude people, the women are generally degraded, among civilised people, they are exalted . . . nothing can exceed the habitual contempt which the Hindus entertain for their women'. James Mill, *The History of British India*, Vol. 2, New York: Chelsea House, 1968, 309–310.

22 Meredith Borthwick, *The Changing Role of Women in Bengal, 1849–1905*, Princeton, NJ: Princeton University Press, 1984, 37.

23 A number of scholars like Lata Mani and Mrinalini Sinha have discussed how Indian women were deprived of any agency in the reform initiatives of the colonial state or the indigenous male elites. For details see Lata Mani, *Contentious Traditions: The Debate on Sati in Colonial India*, Berkeley: University of California Press, 1998; Mrinalini Sinha, 'Gender in the Critiques of Colonialism and Nationalism: Locating the Indian Woman', in Tanika Sarkar and Sumit Sarkar, eds. *Women and Social Reform in Modern India: A Reader*, Indiana: Indiana University Press, 2008; for a detailed critique of patriarchy from Indian feminists' point of view, see Kumkum Sangari and Sudesh Vaid, ed. *Recasting Women: Essays in Indian Colonial History*, New Brunswick, NJ: Rutgers University Press, 1990.

24 Tanika Sarkar, 'Hindu Wife, Hindu Nation: Domesticity and Nationalism in Nineteenth-Century Bengal', in Tanika Sarkar, ed. *Hindu Wife, Hindu Nation: Community, Religion, and Cultural Nationalism*, New Delhi: Permanent Black, 2000, 27–28.

25 Samarpita Mitra, 'The Literary Public Sphere in Bengal: Aesthetics, Culture and Politics, 1905–1939', Unpublished PhD dissertation, University of Syracuse, 2009, Introduction.

26 Borthwick, *The Changing Role of Women*.

27 H. Beverley, *Report on the Census of Bengal, 1872*, Calcutta: Bengal Secretariat Press, 1872, 140.

28 Shib Chunder Deb, *Sisupalan, Part I*, Serampore: Mission Press, 1857, Part II, Calcutta, 1868; Gangaprasad Mukhopadhyay, *Matrisiksa*, Calcutta, 1871.

29 See '*Dhatribidya: Sutikagar* (The Art of Midwifery: Site of Birth)', *Bamabodhini Patrika*, Vol.3, No.52, November 1867, 636.

30 Jayanta Bhattacharya, 'The Genesis of Hospital Medicine in India: The Calcutta Medical College (CMC) and the Emergence of a New Medical Epistemology', *Indian Economic and Social History Review*, Vol.51, No.2, 2014, 231–264; also see Jayanta Bhattacharya, 'Anatomical Knowledge and East-West Exchange', in Deepak Kumar and Raj Sekhar Basu, eds. *Medical Encounters in British India*, New Delhi: Oxford University Press, 2013.

31 'Medical College', *The Asiatic Journal and Monthly Register for British and Foreign India*, December 1837, 240.

32 Moscucci traces the rise of the discipline of obstetrics and gynaecology in nineteenth-century England till the foundation of the Royal

College of Obstetricians and Gynaecologists in 1929. Moscucci Ornella Moscucci, *The Science of Woman: Gynaecology and Gender in England, 1800–1929*, Cambridge: Cambridge University Press, 1990.

33  *Antahpur* was started in 1898 and edited first by Banalata Devi and then by Hemantakumari Chowdury and Kumudini Mitra. It was managed entirely by women and the intended audience was literate middle-class women who regularly contributed to the journal.

  *Bamabodhini Patrika* was perhaps the most important women's magazine that came into circulation in 1863 through the efforts of the liberal Brahmo reformers who took an active interest in championing the cause of female education. The magazine became the most important vehicle of home tutoring or *antahpur siksa* in the nineteenth century. It published important articles on various subjects pertaining to female education such as geography, science, cookery, literature and health. It remained in circulation for several decades.

  *Bangamahila* was started by the principal of a female school for formal education in 1868. It remained in circulation for only two years. Nevertheless, it was published with a view to educating the zenana women and, hence, remains an important source for understanding male perception of women's issues in the nineteenth century.

  *Bangalakshmi* was started in 1924 and continued for a long period. It published matters of moral, religious, scientific and educational importance.

  *Bharati* was edited by Swarnakumari Devi, sister of Rabindranath Tagore. It was a literary magazine of eminence but published important articles on science as well. Apart from *Antahpur*, it was a prominent journal edited by women and was widely circulated for a long period of time. It was one of the longest-running magazines in the colonial times.

  *Paricarika* was started by Girishchandra Sen. It continued for twenty-eight years. It contained essays on child rearing and household management.

34  Amiya P. Sen, *Hindu Revivalism in Bengal, 1872–1905: Some Essays in Interpretation*, Delhi: Oxford University Press, 1993; Kamala Sen, '*Prasuti Mangal* (Maternal Welfare)', *Bangalakshmi*, Vol.5, No.9, August 1931, 701–704.

35  Sarkar, 'Domesticity and Nationalism'. Shastras broadly referred to Hindu scriptures composed in Sanskrit which explained religious and legal systems and ideas which underscored the basis of the Hindu way of life.

36  I have deliberately stuck to the term 'allopathy' throughout the chapter. In a recent illuminating article, Shinjini Das has argued that the term allopathy was not consciously used by the colonial state to propagate western medicine at least till the early part of the nineteenth century. Rather terms such as 'official medicine', 'state medicine' or 'English medicine' were copiously used in official correspondences. The term 'allopathy' was circulated and popularised as the most accepted term for state-sponsored western medicine in Bengal through scientific polemics that became a regular feature of popular print in the second half of the nineteenth century. For details, see Shinjini Das, 'Debating Scientific Medicine: Homeopathy and Allopathy in Late 19th-Century Medical Print in Bengal', in *Medical History*, 2012, Vol.56, No.4, 2012, 463–480.

37 Ghulam Murshid, *Reluctant Debutante: Response of Bengali Women to Modernisation, 1849–1905*, Rajshahi: Sahitya Samsad, 1985. Partha Chatterjee, *Nation and Its Fragments: Colonial and Postcolonial Histories*, New Delhi: Oxford University Press, 1997, 117.

38 A similar argument has been made by Dipesh Chakrabarty. His depiction of the middle-class Bengali patriarch's effort to construct the idea of women as *grihalakshmi* (goddess of home) and *kulalakshmi* (upholder of the family lineage) resonates Partha Chatterjee's 'nationalist resolution of women's question'. Women, according to Chakrabarty, emerged as non-autonomous and non-secular entities in the anti-colonial, nationalist discourse framed by the indigenous elites. For details, see Dipesh Chakrabarty, 'The Difference: Deferral of (A) Colonial Modernity: Public Debates on Domesticity in British Bengal', *History Workshop*, Vol.36, 1993, 1–34.

39 Himani Bannerji, 'Projects of Hegemony: Towards a Critique of Subaltern Studies "Resolution of the Women's Question"', *Economy and Political Weekly*, Vol.35, No.11, March 2000, 902–920. Of late, Charu Gupta has questioned Partha Chatterjee's argument. Gupta's analysis of the reconfiguration of the domestic space in the context of middle-class identity imaginings in colonial Uttar Pradesh refutes Partha Chatterjee's central theoretical formulation. She argues how debates about domesticity and the centrality of women in the private sphere found their way into the public domain as fluidly as debates raised in the material world ruled by the colonisers were constantly made use of by the middle-class men in reconstituting 'home'. For details, see Charu Gupta, *Sexuality, Obscenity and Community: Women, Muslim and the Hindu Public in Colonial India*, New York: Palgrave Macmillan, 2002.

40 For instance, see Anindita Ghosh, *Behind the Veil: Resistance, Women and the Everyday in Colonial South Asia*, London: Palgrave Macmillan, 2008. Also see Malini Bhattacharya and Abhijit Sen, eds. *Talking of Power: Early Writings of Bengali Women from the Mid-nineteenth to the Beginning of the Twentieth Century*, Kolkata: Stree, 2003, Introduction.

41 Antoinette Burton, 'Contesting the Zenana: The Mission to Make Lady Doctors for India, 1874–1885', *The Journal of British Studies*, Vol.35, No.3, 1996, 368–397.

42 Forbes, 'Education to Earn', 140.

43 Engels, 'The Politics of Childbirth', 150.

44 Paul, 'The Uneasy Alliance'. More significantly, Supriya Guha in her extensive research on medicalisation of childbirth in colonial Bengal concluded that 'the medicalisation of childbirth would not have extended to the middle classes with the relative ease with which it did if it were not for the role of medical women'. Guha, 'A History of the Medicalisation of Childbirth', 194.

45 Monica H. Green, 'Gendering the History of Women's Healthcare', *Gender and History*, Vol.20, No.3, 2008, 487–518; Nancy M. Theriot, 'Women's Voices in Nineteenth-Century Medical Discourse: A Step Toward Deconstructing Science', *Signs*, Vol.19, 1993, 1–31.

46 Eliot Friedson, *Professional Powers: A Study of the Institutionalisation of Formal Knowledge*, Chicago: University of Chicago Press, 1988, 16 and 20.

47 Ibid., 35.

48  Sumit Sarkar, *The Swadeshi Movement in Bengal, 1903–1908*, New Delhi: Permanent Black, 2010.

49  Partha Chatterjee, *Nationalist Thought and the Colonial World: A Derivative Discourse*, Second Edition, London: Zed Books, 1993, 11.

50  *Svasthya* started in 1897 and soon established itself as a major vernacular health periodical. It published extensively on plague during plague outbreak in Bombay and Calcutta. It also contained significant articles on social issues related to health.
    *Cikitsa Sammilani* was a prominent journal edited by very eminent medical personalities like Dr Annadacharan Khastagir. It was subscribed by people beyond the pale of medical profession. It contained important writings on allopathy, homeopathy and Ayurveda.

51  Jane Lewis, *The Politics of Motherhood: Child and Maternal Welfare in England, 1900–1939*, London: Croom Helm, 1980. Apart from England, historical research of a similar nature was being conducted in other countries as well. For instance, Philippa Mein Smith has charted the contours of reforms in obstetrics in New Zealand in the interwar period through a detailed focus on the medicalisation of childbirth and the evolution of antenatal care as major themes of analysis. For details, see Philippa Mein Smith, *Maternity in Dispute: New Zealand 1920–1939*, Wellington: Department of Internal Affairs, Historical Publications Branch, 1986.

52  Lewis, *The Politics of Motherhood*, 16.

53  The *Indian Medical Gazette* provides insights into the priorities that guided the colonial government in instituting midwifery education in Bengal, also documenting official view on Indian birthing practices and maternal and infant mortality in the twentieth century.

54  Maneesha Lal, 'The Politics of Gender and Medicine in Colonial India: The Countess of Dufferin Fund', *Bulletin of the History of Medicine*, Vol.68, No.1, Spring 1994, 29–66.

55  A.R. Arney, *The Power and Profession of Obstetrics*, Chicago and London: Chicago University Press, 1982, 8–9.

56  Sean Lang, 'Colonial Compassion and Political Calculation: The Countess of Dufferin and Her Fund', in Poonam Bala, ed. *Contesting Colonial Authority: Medicine and Indigenous Responses in Nineteenth- and Twentieth Century India*, Plymouth: Lexington Books, 2012, 93.

57  Ann Oakley, *The Captured Womb: A History of the Medical Care of Pregnant Women*, Oxford: Basil Blackwell, 1984, 72.

# 1 Scientific mothers and healthy infants

## The birth of a 'Modern-Scientific' discourse in Bengal, 1860s–1900

> No technology carries the force to change institutional arrangements automatically. Nor does a 'scientific advance', by itself, effect change. No technology will gain widespread acceptance and be the basis of reform of culture unless it is introduced into an ideologically fertile social field or unless such a field can be cultivated around it.[1]

The above observation was made by the eminent sociologist W. R. Arney in explaining the evolution of the profession of obstetrics in the West. Arney sought to link the pace of scientific advance in a society with the degree of preparedness displayed by that particular society in welcoming the new scientific paradigm and the structure of knowledge woven around it. Under the impact of colonial rule, Bengal experienced gradual but complex sociocultural transformations in the early nineteenth century that was not merely premised on a linear movement from an indigenous/pre-modern society to a modern one but on a more convoluted interface between the indigenous/traditional and the modern. Yet, certain components of the western civilisation and culture were perceived as agents of progress and, therefore, readily assimilated into the cultural terrain of Bengal. The emergence of western science and its crucial role in shaping middle-class psyche is illustrative of this fact.

The spawning of an entire corpus of critical literature on the history of science and technology has now dubbed western science as the fulcrum of colonial modernity and also the basis for validating colonial domination in India while also pointing out how science evolved into a dominant cultural expression and was fastidiously held on to by the colonised elite in voicing their own hegemonic aspirations to power.[2] The foundation of the Calcutta Medical College (CMC) and the consequent introduction of western medical paradigm in Bengal

are poignant examples of how western medical science was internalised and appropriated in questioning or, at times, subverting existing
parameters of knowledge and permitting the creation of new structures of thought. It is the aim of this chapter to situate the history of
modernisation of childbirth within the boundaries of an 'ideologically
fertile social field' that emerged in response to colonial modernity. The
objective is to understand the extent to which changing sociocultural
milieu facilitated the incorporation of western medical ideas and new
scientific paradigm into the cultural domain of birth. In doing so, the
chapter veers away from extraneous agents like Christian missionaries
and locates the reform of midwifery and birthing practices within an
indigenous domain manoeuvred by the enlightened elites of Bengal.

The spotlight of the chapter being chiefly on the Hindu middle-class
(commonly known as bhadralok) discourse on health, the discussion is
situated at the heart of a self-fashioning project of the bhadralok that
increasingly rendered itself visible in the textual spaces of the vernacular magazines in the late nineteenth century. In a bid to wrest claims to
cultural and political leadership from the colonisers, the middle class
stopped short of altogether renouncing colonial modernity and instead
chose to appropriate it in its own terms. The ensuing struggle to reconstitute its 'national yet modern self'[3] significantly touched upon the
most foundational aspects of social life: the family and the women.
An entire gamut of concerns pertaining to domesticity, conjugality,
health, childbearing and childrearing were beginning to be reconfig-
ured in accordance with the shifting preferences of the middle class.
The chapter seeks to demonstrate how many of the changes effected
by the middle class were driven by modern and scientific sensibilities
that overwhelmingly came to influence bhadralok ideology from the
1830s and 1840s, and acquired greater visibility in the burgeoning
print culture of the 1860s.

The booming print culture in Bengal in the second half of the nineteenth century enabled the constitution of a discursive forum where
the cultural and nationalist imaginings of womanhood were contested,
negotiated and reworked. In this context, Samarpita Mitra has recently
highlighted the critical role of Bengali periodicals in forging an 'idea of
Bengaliness, a particular form of identity articulated in aesthetics and
literary terms, invested with its own distinctive cultural and ideological
project'.[4] Mitra also alluded to the construction of a 'women's sphere'
within the textual space of the magazines as an important constituent
in the ideological formation of this Bengaliness. A close reading of the
women's magazines indicates the centrality of motherhood in redefining womanhood. Elevated notions of motherhood lay at the heart of

patriarchal attempts to discipline, regulate and modernise women as the *janani* (mother) and *grihini* (mistress of the home); it formed a powerful pretext for educating the womenfolk about health science including the essentials of reproductive health.

In the recent researches on print culture and periodicals, the centrality of vernacular health magazines in disseminating medical ideas, promoting health education and determining public opinion on varied aspects of health has largely been overlooked.[5] The contribution of such magazines lay in interpreting crucial social issues in scientific terms in a manner that would appeal to the modern, rational sensibilities of the middle-class readers (men and women).[6] Most importantly, the magazines enunciated a nationalist vision – of a modern discourse on health as the index for national regeneration.[7] However, nationalism at this stage spoke more of Bengaliness than any lofty idea of a pan-Indian nationhood.

The authorship of the earlier articles on midwifery and women's health in vernacular women's magazines is largely obscured. In all probability, they were not compositions by the women medical graduates who emerged as a professional group only after the establishment of the Dufferin Fund in 1885 and more coherently from 1891 onwards.[8] That lends heft to the assumption that the bulk of the essays were written by Bengali male reformers including medical students, particularly the graduates of the vernacular licentiate class of the CMC. Such articles in the women's magazines were also published as translated versions of widely publicised British books on midwifery or extracts from lectures delivered by British obstetricians, for instance, by Dr James Simpson.[9] In magazines such as *Bharati* and *Antahpur* that were managed exclusively by women and came into publication in the 1870s and 1890s, respectively, the writers were invariably literate females from the upper and middle echelons of Bengali society.

## Reconfiguring the family: a rational exercise

In the nineteenth century, the sociocultural context of Bengal was shaped by major transformative strands that had resonances in the West. The emergence of the 'modern' and 'scientific' sensibilities of the Bengalis that rendered itself visible in multivalent forms in the second half of the nineteenth century constituted an unmistakable articulation of the changing perceptions of the newly colonised middle class. Scientific ideas couched in the rhetoric of reason profoundly influenced the bhadralok's approach towards predominant social questions of the time. It underscored the basis for the reconfiguration of the society. The primary social unit of family as conveyed by the notions of domesticity and conjugality was sought to be reconstituted along redefined social and cultural parameters. In the process, pregnancy and childbearing practices as crucial elements of domestic and conjugal life became subjects of a fervent public debate. This was especially in view of the disconcerting reports of infant deaths being published by official sources that attributed loss of infant life to the negligence and irrational practices of the womenfolk. Such ideas were avidly circulated by popular magazines from the 1860s. Long before the nationalist anxieties over the increasing rate of infant and maternal mortality were articulated in press in the interwar years of the twentieth century, a fledgling attempt to modernise existing midwifery practices was made by the liberal reformers in the nineteenth century that had interesting resonances in the nationalist discourse on childbirth in the following century.

The bhadralok or the educated/professional middle class (*madhyabitta shreni*) originated out of the sheer administrative and commercial necessities of an expanding colonial bureaucratic structure in the nineteenth century. Crucial to the colonial vision of creating a subservient middle class as the 'agency of economy and administration' was the introduction of English education into the educational curriculum as the conduit through which European ideologies were meant to be diffused amongst the colonised. The Charles Woods Despatch of 1854 tied English education to the more explicitly secular objective of instilling the values of capital and labour amongst the indigenous population and cull their creative potentials in bolstering the political economy of the colonisers.[10] English educational textbooks sought to project and inculcate the self-proclaimed western qualities of 'rationality', 'manliness', 'physical fitness' and 'progressiveness' against the alleged Indian propensities to be 'superstitious', 'effeminate', 'weakly' and 'decadent'.[11] Such contrived notions of British 'masculinity' as opposed to the much ridiculed 'femininity' of Indians struck deep psychological roots in Indian sensibilities, leading to what Ashish Nandy famously describes as an enduring imagination of modern West as less of a 'geographical and temporal entity' and more of a 'psychological category'.[12]

Induction of the newly emergent middle-class men into the professional sphere of *chakri* or salaried employment was singularly enabled by the introduction of English education in Bengal by the English Education Act of 1835.[13] The Act marked the first major step towards the dissemination of European moral and religious values amongst the Indians through the conduit of English education. Charles Wood's famous Despatch of 1854 went a step ahead in delinking English education from its moral and religious objectives and tying it to the overtly secular motive of furtherance of political economy of the British.[14] The redefined objective was to 'teach the natives of India the marvellous results of the employment of labour and capital, rouse them to emulate us in the development of the vast resources of their country'.[15]

English education and the subsequent entry into the precincts of the colonial offices regulated by strict discipline and 'clock-time' endowed the bhadralok with the consciousness of a modern self.[16] At the same time, the 'routinised' nature of office work generated a sense of estrangement from the traditional mode of existence which was further complicated by subordination to colonial employers and the everyday humiliation that such conditions of employment came to signify. The consequence was a pronounced awareness of the need to retain family as the site for the preservation of traditional social order. Yet, the impact of western education was equally colossal in fashioning a modern, scientific consciousness of the colonised middle class, leading to some of the aspects of traditional cultural practices being questioned and brushed aside as primitive, irrational and backward.

Reason became central to the intellectual pursuits of the Bengali intelligentsia. It was integral to the educational structure that evolved in response to colonial rule in the early nineteenth century, most visible in the curricula of the Hindu College (established in 1817) and similar institutions that sprang up around the same time. The curricula reflected 'strong rationalist bias' and was also 'uniquely secular' for most part of the century.[17] As Gyan Prakash points out:

> New organisations were set up to foster a scientific culture, and existing public bodies included the promotion of science in their activities. Western-educated Indians published tracts on science with or without government patronage, and religious and social reform came to be seen through science's authoritative 'second sight'.[18]

Following the foundation of the Asiatic Society in 1784 as the nucleus for promoting the study of India's 'natural history' and science,[19] a number of socio-religious reform and scientific associations such as the *Brahmo Samaj*, *Tattvabodhini Sabha* and the Society for the Acquisition of General Knowledge came into being, nearly all of them being driven by the pressing motive of evolving 'new forms of thinking and living'.[20] The 'new forms of thinking and living' touched upon the most integral aspects of life embodied in health, domesticity, conjugality, motherhood, childbearing and childrearing.

The western-educated middle class' preoccupation with health became increasingly evident in the 1860s and 1870s, more so in Bengal than in other parts of India. The concern for health was visibly a reaction to the colonial indictment of the Bengalis as 'effeminate'. Tanika Sarkar has traced the root of the Bengali's sense of emasculation to the economic setbacks of the 1830s and 1840s. The low productivity in the 'moribund' delta region of the Ganges and inadequate food supply that was followed by epidemics, recurrent life-threatening fevers and famines substantially contributed towards the structuring of the self-image of a 'frail' Bengali. This awareness of a fragile self lent credence to the idea of effeminacy; manhood, as Sarkar argues, was based on specific 'nature of relationship' to property. The marginalisation of the Bengali entrepreneurs in the modern economic sector from the 1840s by the European agency houses and the Marwaris (a North Indian trading community) and the compulsion of the middle class to work in petty clerical positions in colonial administrative establishments generated a profound sense of emasculation which was further boosted by the Rent Acts of 1859 and 1885. The Rent Acts caused substantial erosion in the power and privileges of the zamindars over the tenants since the Permanent Settlement of 1793.[21] Such setbacks, needless to say, struck at the selfhood and dignity of the middle class that had consistently retained a connection with the land. The consequent sense of decline that came to haunt the middle class for the whole of the nineteenth century was further exacerbated by certain racist and exclusivist policies of the colonial state, as evident in the colonial state's refusal to allow the Bengalis the right to bear arms or hold higher positions in the colonial administrative service, by repeatedly questioning their masculinity.[22]

By the 1850s and 1860s, the English-educated middle class had internalised the British stereotype of an 'effeminate Bengali' and sought to overcome this supposed degeneracy through revival of physical culture.[23] An article entitled 'The revival of National Physical Health' that was published in a leading Bengali magazine *Cikitsa Sammilani* admitted that 'most foreigners and some thinking Indians strongly believe that the people of our country have a frail body and a short lifespan and that is certainly not far from the truth'.[24] The solution proposed was that

> if nutritious food is to make the physique properly strong, then
> it is necessary to inhale enough fresh air into the lungs through

physical activities and proper exercise . . . if the respectable, educated and rich people of our country are prepared to undertake the amount of physical exertion that even an English woman does, one of the major impediments against improvement of their bodily health would be removed.[25]

Following the foundation of the CMC and the new medical culture it fostered through the introduction of anatomy and physiology into the academic curriculum, the mechanisms of body became a critical area of interest in the bhadralok discourse on health.[26] Studies in anatomy gave rise to new knowledge practices that rendered the body as a subject of medical/clinical scrutiny. This was in sharp contrast to the existing pattern of medical education in India that principally centred on medical knowledge being passed from the teacher (known as *Kaviraj* in the *Ayurveda* tradition) to the pupil and the latter mastering the classic medical texts written in Sanskrit and preparing medicine under the guidance of the Kaviraj.[27] Therefore, the study of anatomy when introduced as part of the medical curriculum at the Medical College had deeper implications in terms of how health was beginning to be perceived by bhadralok on a medical–scientific basis.

Up to the 1860s, the colonial officials chiefly concerned themselves with diseases that fatally affected the army and the European community. A Royal Commission to Enquire into the Sanitary State of the Army in India was appointed in 1859. The Commission, however, did also make investigation into the health and diseases of the general native Indian population.[28] The health of the Indian population did not usually figure in the official colonial health policy except during the outbreaks of epidemics such as cholera, smallpox and plague that compelled state intervention from time to time. Yet from the 1860s itself, thanks to the profound sense of emasculation haunting the bhadralok and the new forms of knowledge introduced by the Medical College, the Bengali middle class found itself examining the mechanisms of body and ways to secure personal health. Voicing such concerns further in the 1880s, *Cikitsa Sammilani* lamentingly pointed towards a state of existence of the Bengalis in which, 'diseases like malaria, filaria or goitre are rampant, the germs enter the body and affect the blood and the bone marrow, which in turn delimits physical strength and virility'.[29]

The gradual reformulation of existing health practices amongst the bhadralok was evident in the print from the 1860s when medical publications in Bengal proliferated. Such reformulations mostly refrained from overt association with western medical discourse and

were overwhelmingly projected as the modified and simplified rendi-
tions of the indigenous Ayurveda tradition. Such writings constituted
a distinct genre within the huge corpus of medical writings that were
published in this period.[30] To cite an instance, the composition of
one of the earliest health manuals entitled *Sharirik Svasthya Bidhan*
(A Treatise on Physical Health) (1862) was inspired, according to its
author, by the presumed dearth of medical literature in Bengali language that would provide access to the supposedly 'rich' repertoire
of Sanskrit-based Ayurveda medical tradition otherwise inaccessible
for the lay readers.[31] Hence, *Sharirik Svasthya Bidhan*, being written
in lucid Bengali language, propounded health principles that were
designed to regulate the daily habits of people, within the framework
of Ayurveda medical discourse. It emphasised a balanced and nutritious diet, breathing fresh air, drinking pure water and doing physical
exercise and also prompted a certain 'code of conduct' for women
to be observed during menstruation.[32] While the instructions had
nothing overtly western about them, the concern of the author that
men and women be enlightened about certain vital aspects of their
health was a manifestation of the deepening middle-class interest in
the mechanisms of the body; it was, as mentioned earlier, the consequence of a paradigmatic shift caused by the introduction of anatomy
at the Medical College.

The importance of securing personal physical health was reiterated
in various women's magazines of the time. Being usually composed
by male writers the ideas encapsulated in such writings were clearly
tantamount to patriarchal injunctions, a subtle yet pervasive way to
discipline the everyday lives of women. The very first volume of the
popular women's magazine *Bamabodhini Patrika* which was published in 1864 accommodated an elaborate section on health under
the title *Svasthyaraksha*. *Svasthyaraksha* constituted a series of prescriptive essays that highlighted cleanliness, disciplined lifestyle and
balance between work and rest as integral to good health.[33] A series of
articles entitled *Sharirik Svasthyabidhan* ('Rules of Physical Health')
that appeared in *Bamabodhini Patrika* in 1867 endorsed an entire
range of health care principles that further reinforced the notions of a
sanitised self.[34] The crucial feature of the series was, however, the prescriptions on 'proper' mode of entertainment for women and prohibi-
tions on indulgence in obscene gossips, signifying strong patriarchal
ardour for regulating female behaviour.[35]

In the 1870s the broader sociopolitical context in Bengal was
shaped by frenzied propensities to valorise the history, religion and
spiritual tradition of the Hindus, often to the point of 'chauvinism'

and 'cultural bigotry'. However, as Amiya Sen reminds us the essence of this 'cultural revivalism' did not really lie in reviving Hindu tradition per se but in the tendency to attach 'disproportionate importance' to certain aspects of tradition as compared to others.[36] It was the outcome of a series of blatantly discriminatory and racist policies of the colonial regime between the 1860s and the 1890s that resulted in increasing disenchantment of the colonised elites with the emancipatory and progressive capacities of colonial governance.[37]

The revivalist spirit permeated the vernacular literature including medical writings and had interesting resonances in the reformulation of gender relations in the period. In the 1880s the Bengali bhadralok's preoccupation with health acquired new dimensions. Of all the reasons cited for the supposed frailty of the Bengalis, child marriage and premature consummation leading to early pregnancies and debilitating diseases amongst mothers and children formed intense subjects of discussion in the reflective debates of the time. Quite a few medical texts on midwifery appropriated the dominant revivalist mood of the time in interpreting the evils of child marriage from both social and medical perspectives. An illustrative example is perhaps Haranath Ray's *Dhatri-sikkha Samgraha* (Midwife's Vade-Mecum) published in 1887.[38] In an overtly Hindu revivalist tone, Ray traced the origin of the 'decadent', 'irrational' institution of child marriage in the 'tyrannical' phase of Muslim rule, thus denying its origin in the Vedic age when this practice was claimed to have been entirely absent. He asserted that the lecherous disposition of the Muslim ruling elites compelled the Hindus to marry off their daughters at a young age in order to preserve their chastity. Ray condemned child marriage in both social and medical terms: in social terms, by tying it up with other ills such as child widowhood and lack of emotional attachment between the child bride and groom; in medical terms by illuminating the debilitating impact of early/premature maternity on the future of the race.[39] He argued that early menarche in Hindu women followed by early consummation (*garbhadhan*) and pregnancy resulted in the gradual weakening of the Hindu race. If the law of 'Evolution' was to be believed, Hindu race would, in no time, be wiped off the face of the earth.[40]

Haranath Ray's text was therefore conveniently woven around the revivalist sentiment in critiquing child marriage as a practice encouraged by the fear of Muslims. A more persuasive strand of the child marriage debate and also the one that hogged the limelight in the last decade of the nineteenth century was the glorification of the custom as an intrinsic aspect of Hindu tradition and, consequently, infallible on religious grounds. Tanika Sarkar has argued how the reigning conservatism of the revivalist era caused the bhadralok to redirect focus from the public sphere as the arena for the 'test of manhood' to the family as 'an enterprise to be administered, an army to be led, a state to be governed'.[41] Consequently, conjugality in the sense of being the 'loving, willed surrender' of the Hindu wife to the husband became the key principle for the administration of family and assertion of 'native' masculinity. It was perhaps the only viable way to compensate for the subordination in the world outside. Mrinalini Sinha has reinforced Sarkar's argument by demonstrating how the body of Bengali females became a site for the assertion of 'native masculinity' by the revivalist nationalists whose complicity in the politics of colonial masculinity purged nationalist politics of its emancipatory possibilities. It also accounted for the 'curious' silence of the women's magazines on the Age of Consent controversy throughout the period of agitation.[42]

The Age of Consent Bill that was introduced in the Legislative Assembly by Sir Andrew Scoble in January 1891 raised the age of consent for consummation for Indian girls from ten to twelve. While the government was initially paranoid about introducing any new legislation, it eventually yielded to the reformist pressure. The Bill generated a protest of unprecedented enormity in Bengal compared to the rest of India.[43] The revivalists, who constituted the chief opponents of the Bill, alleged that the raising of the age of sexual consummation from ten to twelve violated the *garbhadhan* (consummation) ceremony which constituted one of the major ten rituals of the Hindus.[44] It was tantamount to tampering with *Shastric* injunctions and the sacrosanct religious practices of the Hindus. In the face of the massive conservative backlash, the voices of the doctors and liberal reformers arguing in favour of the Bill were enfeebled and eventually drowned. Yet in hindsight, the voices of the opponents of the Bill proved equally ephemeral. As Amiya Sen has aptly argued, the Age of Consent issue was more of a 'symbolic' one 'on the basis of which political strength or preparedness could be reasonably tested' as people quickly moved on to 'newer channels of self-expression'.[45] Child marriage continued to engage the attention of medical men and liberal social reformers in the 1890s and more powerfully from the early twentieth century.[46] It elicited critical reactions from the bhadramahila at the turn of the century and featured prominently in the Indian feminist discourse in the 1920s and 1930s. The roots of Bengali women's awareness about health and other social factors conditioning their lives lay in the female education movement that emerged as part of the social reform movement in nineteenth-century Bengal.

## Educating the Bhadramahila in health science

The complex process of the reconfiguration of bhadralok identity in nineteenth-century Bengal placed the question of the 'degraded' status of women at the core of its reformist/modernising self-improvement agenda. The colonial indictment of the debased conditions of Hindu women as an unmistakable sign of the inferiority of Hindu civilisation struck at the crux of the selfhood of the western-educated intellectuals. It triggered collaborative efforts between the social reformers and the colonial state in putting an end to certain decadent social norms responsible for the low status of women. Notable reforms included the campaign against Sati and its subsequent abolition through state legislation (1829) and the Widow Remarriage Act of 1856. The more enduring reformist initiative, however, lay in promoting female education that underscored a sustained basis for the modernisation of women, albeit within the constrictive framework of Hindu patriarchal notions of nationhood. Such notions, as Partha Chatterjee has argued, symbolically associated women with the 'inner' 'spiritual' realm of home in which dwelt the true essence of Hindu nation. Thus, woman was to be educated and elevated and yet placed firmly in the traditional strictures of family and home. Judith Walsh has further argued that the bhadralok's exposure to English education and modern work ambience necessitated a reformulation of the role of women in a bid to ensure greater compatibility between the home (*griha*) and the world (*bahir*). The re-imagination of woman as an amalgamation of a romantic partner and 'family-oriented' daughter-in-law and also a dextrous housewife was in reality a foreign idea. The idea was, however, stripped of its foreignness and linked to the traditional world of the Bengalis in reconstituting a new inner sphere of home.[47]

While female education was unequivocally acknowledged as the most effective way to elevate women from their debased state of being, the nature and content of education became a site of heated contestation. The long-standing deliberations on the content of the curriculum for female education from the 1840s onwards reflected the deep-seated concerns of both the bhadralok and the colonial officials to ensure the enhancement and refinement of 'feminine' sensibilities of women. In a lecture delivered at the Bethune Society in 1863, Kumar Harendra Krishna, the *Maharajah* of Hathwah,[48] clearly spelt out the objectives of female education in the following words:

> Our need is to devise such a system of education for the Hindu female as will make her an agreeable companion, a good mother,

an intellectual and loving wife and an excellent housewife. We want her to be well grounded in the moral virtues recognised by the civilisation of which we are the co-sharers, and to possess those superior mental accomplishments which enable the wife to serve as a solace to the husband in his brightest and darkest moments, the mother to undertake or at least superintend the early instruction of her child, and the lady of the house to provide those sweet social comforts idealised by the talismanic word – home.[49]

This was to be attained through training women in subjects like needlework, embroidery with a smattering of grammar, geography and mathematics.[50] Despite pure science and mathematics being marginalised in the curriculum, the apparently exalted position accorded to women as wives and mothers led to a minimum knowledge of health science being endorsed as crucial for the rational management of domesticity and motherhood. In the process, the roles of the new woman or bhadramahila were more vividly spelt out.

The *Bamabodhini Patrika* which was started in 1863 by the Brahmo leaders for educating the Bengali middle-class women played a pivotal role in crystallising the image of bhadramahila. The overwhelming challenge faced by these leaders was 'how to be both in line with Western-oriented modernisation in which women were *to know of* the outside world and in line with indigenous tradition in which they were *not to be* a part of it' (emphasis original).[51] *Bamabodhini* addressed the dilemma through instituting *antahpur siksa* or home tutoring. As the 'main purveyor of antahpur schooling', *Bamabodhini* began to publish syllabus for home tutoring in the 1860s. Amongst the subjects mentioned in the syllabus such as Bengali literature, grammar, elementary knowledge of geography, arithmetic and science, preservation of health (*svasthya raksha*) also featured regularly.[52] It also published educative and prescriptive essays on domesticity, childbearing and childrearing under the titles of *Ramanir Kartabya* ('Duties of a Woman'), *Dhatribidya* ('Art of Midwifery') and *Sisu Palan* ('Infant Rearing') in the second half of the nineteenth century.

Reordering home was central to the reconstitution of domesticity. In stressing upon cleanliness, hygiene and order that clearly echoed Victorian ideals of domesticity, the new middle-class discourse sought to discard older traditions of household management that allegedly trivialised the importance of 'order' and 'hygiene'. To offer an example, in a series of articles entitled *Ramanir Kartabya*, the author outlined the role of a bhadramahila in reordering her home under three major headings, *Bas Bhaban* (Drawing Room), *Shajya Bhaban* (Bedroom) and *Bhandar Bhaban* (Kitchen). The bhadramahila was advised to keep the food and other edible products in labelled containers for greater clarity and order; to keep the bedroom airy, clean, properly dusted and well furnished and to put the pillows, bed cover and bed sheets under sun and also to keep out mosquitoes.[53]

By the same token, health science was perceived by reformers as a crucial element of female education, healing and nursing being considered as 'natural' feminine attributes.[54] As stated earlier, in the fervent debate on the scope of female education in mid-nineteenth-century Bengal, there was a general disapproval of girls being instructed in mathematics and science.[55] Yet, knowledge of health science and remedies for minor diseases was deemed essential for bhadramahila in her role as a *grihini* or *grihakatri* (females in charge of household management). A writer's lamentations in *Bamabodhini* on the ignorance of the contemporary women in matters of health provide a typical example. He stated ruefully:

> Not very long ago, the womenfolk of our country knew medical cures for a variety of ailments. Even today, women living in the mufassils or the older women of the city are seen to treat the minor ailments of girls and boys; it used to be an educational job like any other household chore. If any member of the household fell ill, instead of calling the doctor in the first instance, the mistress of the household would try to alleviate the pain by applying her tried and tested medicines and even succeeded in eradicating it in many cases. But in the present times, girls are acquiring education in the schools but are not learning anything on this subject and nobody is paying heed to this.[56]

Many of such writings in the 1870s and 1880s coalesced around the image of the bhadramahila as the repository of 'traditional'/indigenous medical knowledge reflecting the dominant revivalist mood of the times. The reassertion of the value of traditional medicines presumed the unsuitability of state-sponsored western allopathic medicines in addressing and remedying indigenous health problems. The only interesting exception was homeopathy which despite being of German in origin readily gained acceptance in the Bengali popular psyche. As scholars have pointed out, the proliferation of homeopathic tracts on myriad aspects of health hinged on the promise for inexpensive self-cure. The middle-class penchant for homeopathic treatment as opposed to allopathy that was identified as the 'state medicine' or scornfully referred to as 'English medicine' sat well with the prevailing cultural revivalist temperament of the time. Despite operating outside the orbit of state legislation, homeopathy was popularised largely through bhadralok elite endeavours and private enterprises and, in the process, was thoroughly indigenised.[57] For instance, the author of an essay entitled *Garhasthya Cikitsa Pranali* ('Methods of Home Treatment'), published in *Bamabodhini Patrika* in 1871, asserted that:

> Those women who are acquiring education in a slightly improved manner can study the translated versions of the Homeopathy medical books under the supervision of a competent and learned person. I can state with some courage that a little knowledge of homeopathy medicine can prove beneficial to them.[58]

Notwithstanding such negotiations with indigenous medical ideas, certain epistemic aspects of allopathic medicine were internalised in formulating a modern and scientific approach to vital areas associated with health. Such improvised notions were progressively disseminated to the women.

One such area was the knowledge of human anatomy. From the early 1870s rudimentary knowledge of the functioning of the human body was being diffused through the pages of women's journals. While articles entitled *Sharirik kriya* ('Functions of the Body') featuring regularly in *Bamabodhini Patrika* took the lead, lesser-known magazines such as *Bangamahila* ('Women of Bengal') also did not lag behind in enlightening the female readers on the anatomical and biological details of the human body. A series of articles entitled *Svasthya Raksha* ('Preserving the Health') which appeared in 1875 provided detailed anatomical and physiological descriptions of the human body such as the functions of breathing (respiration), blood circulation, digestion, interspersed with diagrams of the intestine, lungs and the heart, explaining the position of the valves and the arteries. It contained elaborate descriptions of the functioning of the human brain including the functions of the five senses.[59] Such instructions on the anatomy and physiology of human body were being derived from the clinical/scientific paradigms of western medical science.

The drive to educate women in health science was, therefore, suffused with complex and contradictory meanings. It allowed a reimagination of woman as the storehouse of indigenous medical knowledge in consonance with her newly defined role as the preserver of the sanctified domain of household, uncontaminated by colonialism. That implied retention of the older forms of knowledge at the cost of marginalising the new paradigm introduced by state-sponsored western medical science. Yet the very attempt at educating women in human anatomy and assigning them the task of modernising birthing practices at home (as the next section will demonstrate) signified privileging the newer system of knowledge over the older ones. It indicated the growing faith of a section of the middle class in the superiority of western medical knowledge over existing medical traditions. The break between the older and newer forms of knowledge was seldom sharp, being mostly based on reconciliation between the two. What was perhaps more central to the constitution and dissemination of knowledge was the rhetoric of science and the way it influenced the interpretation of existing forms of knowledge.

## The physiology and anatomy of birth

In the emerging discourse on the centrality of 'svasthya raksha' (preservation of health) in the regeneration of the Bengalis, the female-controlled domain of midwifery gradually surfaced as one of the crucial areas of concern in the second half of the nineteenth century. Concern for the loss of infant life due to 'neonatal tetanus' (locally referred to in Bengal and in Bengali magazines as *pechoyepawa*) brought the allegedly barbaric practices of the dhais and ignorant womenfolk of the Bengali household under scrutiny. The composition of one of the earliest treatises on infant rearing in 1857 was prompted by the alleged ignorance of the Bengali women of the principles of childrearing resulting in unnecessary loss of infant life.[60] It was ruefully pointed out in *Bamabodhini* that despite the birth of a child being extremely desired in a Bengali household – with prospective parents engaging in intense prayers, meditation and ritual penance – the irrational practices and the unhygienic surroundings of birth led to an unfortunate waste of infant life.[61]

Disconcerting reports on infant mortality were published in newspapers from the 1870s. In 1876, for instance, the *Amrita Bazar Patrika*, quoting a report compiled by an IMS official, revealed:

> Of every thousand Hindu children born about 1875, there died 596 within a year, and of the Mahomedans, no less than 735; while the annual average of the latter was 598 . . . *a native child born healthy in the town has a chance of life considerably less than that of a person attacked with cholera.*(emphasis original)[62]

Public anxieties over infant mortality were further accentuated by official reports, especially the census reports from 1881 onwards, which revealed high infant and maternal mortality rates.[63] The census of 1881 observed in an alarmist tone that 'out of every 1000 infants born in Calcutta, 488 die before they reach the age of 12 months . . . it is not incredible when the circumstances are remembered in India, and especially in a crowded town like Calcutta, surround the infant during its first few days of life'.[64] Competing explanations of the causes, symptoms and treatment of *pechoyepawa* (neonatal tetanus) according to the prevalent allopathy, homeopathy and Ayurveda traditions were published in *Cikitsa Sammilani* from 1886 onwards.[65] Such publications reached a wider reading community beyond the pale of medical profession.[66] Reforming midwifery was also perceived as an important step towards creating an educated mother as an integral component of the process of modernisation. The Bengali middle-class perception of existing midwifery practices being problematic was partly a response to the concerns voiced by the women Christian missionaries charged with the responsibility of educating the women of the antahpur/zenana.[67] Also, following the opening of a Bengali class at the CMC in 1864, there was an increased awareness of the medical significance of midwifery amongst the male students, most of whom belonged principally to the bhadralok class.[68] A shining instance was the demand raised by these students in 1866 for theoretical and practical training in midwifery, resulting in the appointment in 1868 of a 'Native Sub-Assistant Surgeon' as the teacher of midwifery, on a permanent basis.[69] While it is doubtful that the newly trained doctors immediately penetrated the zenana with their knowledge, the incident, no doubt, marks the eagerness of the bhadralok to appropriate the new paradigms of knowledge on midwifery offered by western medical science. However, in the absence of direct access into the female spheres, the bhadralok invented an alternative strategy of transferring the new knowledge to the bhadramahila through the prevalent form of 'home tutoring' introduced by *Bamabodhini*.

The series of articles entitled *Dhatribidya* ('Art of Midwifery') and *Sisu Palan* ('Child Rearing') which began to appear in *Bamabodhini Patrika* from 1866 and continued till the early 1870s embodied the earliest initiatives of the reformist section of the bhadralok to introduce western medical ideas into the secluded quarters of zenana or antahpur, at least two decades before the colonial state took an interest in it through the foundation of the Dufferin Fund in 1885. Being one of the longest-running women's magazines in Bengal from 1863 to 1922, *Bamabodhini* enjoyed a wide and popular readership.[70] *Dhatribidya* and *Sisu Palan* were written with the aim of introducing middle-class women to the physiology and anatomy of their own body and to a scientific understanding of the functioning of the reproductive system, so that false notions associated with parturition could be dispelled and a more rational understanding of pregnancy and childbirth based on the new information be introduced.

One of the earliest articles in the *Dhatribidya* series published in *Bamabodhini Patrika* in 1867 outlined the imperatives for starting the series in the following words:

> The prevalent superstition and ignorance among the pregnant women have resulted in a number of mishaps. Therefore, they should be made aware of their duties during pregnancy. To attain a sound knowledge of midwifery it is essential to learn about the functions of the abdomen, pelvis and the change in the position of the foetus in the uterus. However, it is illogical to write down such details in Bamabodhini. Those aspects of midwifery which the women readers will not feel embarrassed to read will be discussed here.[71]

The author, therefore, set the parameters of the knowledge to be delivered to the women readers. This series of articles later straddled an extensive range of subjects relating to pregnancy such as biological details of the process of pregnancy, care of pregnant women (earliest hints on antenatal care), management of labour and care of the mother and the infant after delivery.[72] All of these had interesting resonances in the constitution of a medical discourse on childbirth following the incorporation of midwifery in the medical curriculum of the CMC in 1841. The essays were also testimony to the fact that the knowledge of the anatomy of female body was a male preserve in nineteenth-century Bengal as in many other parts of the world, female body being an object of male scientific scrutiny. The knowledge of female anatomy was, however, to be disseminated to the women to the extent that would enlighten them about certain scientific aspects of pregnancy and teach them measures to safeguard the life of the infant in the interest of the family and nation.

The earlier essays of the *Dhatribidya* series began with critiquing the site of birth. One of the earliest in the series blamed the prevalent 'superstition' and 'ignorance' for preventing childbirth from taking place within the main precincts of the household. This allegedly led to the construction of *sutikagriha* (place of birth) in that corner of the house which was the filthiest and the most ill-ventilated, causing irreparable damage to the life of the infant. Thus, it was advised that the room which was 'spacious, airy with windows open on the south' be selected as the ideal site of birth.[73] The recurrence of the denunciation of *sutikagriha* in both bhadralok and colonial writings led to initiatives being taken later by the Dufferin Fund to implement hospitalisation of birth by opening a country-wide network of female-run hospitals, a trend that falteringly gained acceptance in the next century. Further, the image of *sutikagriha* as the abode of sickness and post-pregnancy complications acquired renewed centrality in the public debates on maternal and infant mortality in Bengal in the interwar years.

In the later essays of the *Dhatribidya* series, the spotlight shifted from the sociocultural settings of birth to the physiological details of labour. Women were taught to recognise three types of labour: normal labour, delayed labour and abnormal labour. Each of the types was defined briefly and the possibilities of danger to both the mother and the child in case of abnormal labour were spelt out. The duties of the dhais in each of the three stages were also vividly outlined. However, the idea of childbirth as essentially a natural process remained dominant and continued to be reiterated in such discussions. Thus, the author of one such essay concluded:

> The miraculous power of God is reflected in the way the uterus reverts back to its position immediately after the birth of the child. Labour pain cannot be compared with any other pain because it is natural and goes away naturally and quickly. No other pain disappears so quickly on its own.[74]

At the same time, the possibilities of 'abnormality' disrupting the natural process of birth also came to be recognised. The simultaneous focus on the physiological nature of birth and the abnormal aspects of it represented the first signs of problematisation and to some extent pathologisation of midwifery. In an essay entitled *Dhatrir Kartabya* ('Duties of a Dhai') under the *Dhatribidya* series, the author began by acknowledging:

> the way the foetus grows and gains strength within the uterus under divine dispensation, the dhai is not seen to have a weighty role to perform in the entire process. But in whatever little is left for the dhai to do, if she is inexperienced, dangerous consequences may follow which may cause death to both mother and the child.[75]

Despite admonishing the dhai for her unclean and unscientific ways, he eventually bestowed her with the crucial responsibility of examining the parturient women. The dhai had to examine: first, whether the head of the foetus was likely to appear first or any other part of the foetal body; second, the position of the foetus in the uterus; third, the proportion between the pelvis of the mother and the head of the foetus; fourth, the position of the foetal heart; and lastly, the shape and weight of the abdomen.[76] If the mother shied away from giving in to the examination, it was the duty of the dhai to convince her of the utility of such examinations. Here, it is relevant to mention that the concern with 'the proportion between the pelvis of the mother and the head of the foetus' underscored the faint beginnings of a medical approach that emphasised the identification of any possibilities of disproportion as the means to distinguish normal/physiological birth from abnormal/pathological ones.[77] It paved the way for pelvimetry (measuring the size of the pelvis) to be incorporated as a vital component of the professionalised obstetrics during mid-twentieth century. It is, therefore, significant that such ideas found expression in Bengali popular print in as early as the 1860s.

Notwithstanding the frequent denunciation of the dhais in reformist discourse they were deemed as indispensable in Indian birthing practices. In the failure to dislodge them altogether, the only viable option was to instruct them to adopt a regulated and informed approach in handling the three stages of labour. Frequent examinations by them of the pregnant woman and the forcible extraction of the foetal head were warned against and labelled as barbaric. The simultaneous denigration and inclusion of the dhais in the birthing practices in the mid-nineteenth century was part of a complex attempt of the colonised elite to reconcile tradition with newly received scientific ideas from the West. However, much of what was written for the enlightenment of the dhais was often aimed at familiarising the middle-class women with the medical aspects of birth and also making them aware of the unhygienic and unscientific nature of the work performed by the dhais.[78]

*Bamabodhini Patrika* gradually transcended the limits it had set for itself in educating women on the scientific aspects of midwifery. In 1872, an essay entitled *Matrigarbha o Garbhasisu* ('Mother's Womb and the Foetus Within') contained colourful diagrammatic representation of the evolutionary stages of foetal growth inside the mother's womb.[79] Other contemporary journals like *Bharati* too devoted a few pages towards explaining the scientific ways of managing midwifery in Bengal.[80]

By the 1880s, pamphlets written in lucid Bengali language on the science of reproduction by Bengali medical men were proliferating which were addressed to the dhais and the Bengali middle-class readers.[81] For instance, Jadunath Mukherji's *Dhatrisiksa* ('Training the Dhais') published in 1867 aimed to educate both the prospective mother and the dhai in the science of midwifery.[82] Dr Annada Charan Khastagir's 'A Treatise on the Science and Practice of Midwifery with Diseases of Children and Women', which was written in 1868, devoted for the first time a chapter on the diagrammatic illustrations of surgical instruments like forceps, fillets and vectis and described their history and functions in childbirth.[83] Slightly later in the 1880s, Khirodaprosad Chattopadhyay's *Dhatribidya*, a translated version of Dr Playfair's popular book on midwifery, also delineated the surgical aspects of birth.[84] It is not hard to guess that such medical texts rarely found readership amongst the womenfolk of the zenana.[85] Yet as Chapter 2 will argue, such publications substantially contributed towards recasting midwifery along scientific lines.

Midwifery was inextricably bound up with infant rearing (*sisu palan*) which encompassed a wide variety of activities from infant feeding and infant diseases to more profound questions of the moral upbringing of the children. Infant rearing, therefore, required an equally enlightened and refined approach. As early as in 1857, Shib Chunder Deb wrote a treatise entitled *Sisu Palan* on the physiological treatment of infancy which was acknowledged to have been based on Dr Andrew Combe's *Treatise on the Physiological and Moral Management of Infancy*.[86] The second part of the book that was published in 1868 dealt at length with the moral upbringing of children. *Bamabodhini Patrika* published a series of articles entitled *Sisu Palan* in the form of a dialogue between husband and wife in order to ensure greater intelligibility amongst the women readers. Most of such instructive pamphlets which continued to inundate the printing world in the second half of the nineteenth century had strong reverberations of Victorian ideals of motherhood and child rearing. As Meredith Borthwick has demonstrated, the Bengali middle-class discourse on breastfeeding with its insistence on feeding in regulated quantities at 'fixed' times was an outright emulation of the Victorian ideal of 'clockwork functioning' of the household which the bhadralok had substantially internalised in the second half of the nineteenth century.[87] Women were expected to know the physical and mental state of the infant and equip themselves with adequate knowledge of various medicines and treatments for minor disorders.[88]

Despite the discussion in this chapter being chiefly on Hindu bhadralok's transforming perceptions of childbirth practices in the light of received ideas from the West, it is worthwhile to mention that the Muslim middle class also displayed genuine interest in modernising childbearing and childrearing practices. Such trends were amply evident in the manuals written by reformist Muslim men and women towards the end of the nineteenth century. Recent researches have questioned the age-old perception of colonial ethnographers and historians that Muslims were economically depressed under colonial rule and that they remained resistant to western modernity and progress.[89] As Sonia Nishat Amin argues, in the case of Bengal, there was a distinct modernist consciousness amongst a section of Bengali Muslims, mostly men in government jobs from the second half of the nineteenth century. Their agenda of reform which included elevating the social status of women was driven by the dual desires to prove themselves to the colonial rulers and to the more advanced Hindu community. Though slightly later, the Hindu bhadralok discourse on motherhood and childrearing found its way into the writings of Muslim liberal reformers including that of Begum Rokeya Sakhawat Hossain. Rokeya assumed an important role in promoting female education and popularising western model of childcare.[90] However, how many middle-class Muslim women adopted the western model of childcare is not clear from Amin's study. As Chapter 3 will demonstrate, lower-class Muslim women remained trapped in purdah which, in the perception of colonial public health officials, had a bearing on their health and adversely affected infant and maternal mortality figures.

The preceding discussion highlighted the factors that transformed the sociocultural milieu of Bengal in the late nineteenth century. It was now more receptive to western medical ideas that gradually began to find entry into what was once a culturally controlled and female-guarded domain of midwifery. It highlighted the proclivities of a section of the middle class towards appropriating western medical knowledge into the sociocultural fabric of their everyday lives. Outwardly, such trends paved the way for a Bengali woman, Kadambini Basu, to study medicine at the CMC in 1883 even before female medical education had gained formal recognition through the foundation of the Dufferin Fund (1885). Kadambini was, however, vilified by the otherwise conservative Bengali society which was more keen on educating its womenfolk in health science within the confines of the zenana than situating her in the professional public sphere ruled by men. Nonetheless, Kadambini set the trend of female medical education in Bengal which acquired further momentum with the establishment of the Dufferin Fund in 1885.[91]

Notwithstanding the influx of western medical ideas into the antahpur, the actual conditions of birth remained largely unaltered in the second half of the nineteenth century. Women's reproductive health was still on the fringes of direct official concern. The real woman so far was merely the recipient of scientific ideas on pregnancy and infant rearing but still remained outside the purview of medical scrutiny by the medical profession except in few exceptional cases. The high infant and maternal mortality cited in the censuses of 1871 and 1881 constituted strong evidence of the limited success attained in modifying the conditions of childbirth. Sporadic endeavours made by the colonial state to train the native dhais in the 1870s and 1880s often crumbled. The government realised that

> the scope of the experiment should not be confined solely to cases of actual childbirth in the bulk of which probably very little professional knowledge is wanted, but that it should extend also to the diagnosis and treatment of special female diseases. . . . Native women especially of the upper classes from their confined and secluded lives are liable to attacks to this class of diseases and in which they absolutely refuse to place themselves under the treatment of medical men though they would gladly resort to trained midwives.[92]

Around this time, a medical missionary Miss Elizabeth Beilby was requested by the Maharani of Punna to ask Queen Victoria to rescue the sick women of India through proper medical attention. Acting upon Miss Beilby's account, the Queen advised Lady Dufferin – who was ready to set her foot in India along with her newly appointed Viceroy husband Lord Dufferin – that something be done to bring medical aid to the women in India. The advice was tinged with a subtle reference to the 'significant political benefits' that such an endeavour could bring to the colonial government and 'cast it in a benevolent light'.[93] Also the abundance of women doctors in Britain and lack of professional opportunity there due to the dogged resistance of the British male-dominated medical establishment made it convenient for the Queen to permit the women doctors to practise in India where the medical education of women was still in a rudimentary stage.[94] Lady Dufferin's initiative led to the foundation of the 'National Association for supplying female medical aid to the women of India' in 1885, popularly known as the Countess of Dufferin Fund.

Founded under the aegis of the colonial state without being directly under its control,[95] the Dufferin fund was the first major institutionalised step towards imparting medical training to female doctors, nurses and midwives, and providing medical relief to the *purdah-nashin* (secluded) women through female hospitals, dispensaries and trained midwives in the zenana. Notwithstanding the initial success of the Fund partly ascribable to the financial support and enthusiasm of the affluent indigenous elites, its effectiveness in triggering the process of medicalisation of childbirth was rather stultified in Bengal. The reasons are twofold: first, the sustained opposition by the traditional dhais to learn western methods of midwifery[96] and second, the unpopularity of the zenana hospitals in Bengal.[97] Subsequent attempts such as that made by Lady Curzon in 1901 to retrain the dhais through the Victoria Memorial Scholarship Fund crumbled in the face of sustained reluctance of the dhais. Yet, as the next section will show, much had been achieved in the realm of ideas. The booming print culture in late nineteenth-century Bengal that educated women and enabled the dissemination of western scientific and medical ideas into the zenana also, in significant ways, led to educated bhadramahila voicing their own perception of critical social issues integral to their social and biological being. It launched the platform on which future debates on women's deteriorating social and biological status were effectively held in the twentieth century, crystallising feminist agendas for the subsequent decades.

## The response of the Bhadramahila

An analysis of the women's writings in the popular women's magazines of the late nineteenth and early twentieth centuries reveals divergent patterns of thoughts on a complex gamut of issues pertaining to domesticity, childbearing, childrearing and women's health which went under the titles of *Grihe Ramanir Kartabya*, *Sutikagrihe Prasutir Susrusa*, *Santan Palanand and Bharat Mahilar Svasthya*, respectively. Early women's magazines like *Bamabodhini Patrika*, *Bangamahila*, etc., which were entirely run by Bengali male reformers of a liberal disposition, accommodated women writers' views on domestic and conjugal matters. Such writings were, however, circumscribed by the sociocultural predilections of the patriarchy. Ghulam Murshid has highlighted the limited nature of Bengali women's response to social reform which, according to him, was a consequence of lack of understanding of certain economic and legal rights such as the right to property and marriage laws. Freedom, according to Murshid, was understood by Bengali women as improvement of their degraded social position and not as 'emancipation' or 'liberation' in terms of economic independence or sexual liberty.[98] Himani Bannerji has, however, argued that the very participation of women in the print culture of the nineteenth and twentieth centuries enabled them to 'contribute to this formative process of their social subjectivities and agencies'[99] even though the dichotomous nature of this participation alternating between collaboration with patriarchal ideas and resisting them at the same time was very evident at all times. In the process, women emerged as both 'resisting agent and collaborator' of the patriarchal order.[100] The contradictory trends were abundantly manifest in the educated women's writings, for instance, in the simultaneous exaltation of the patriarchal injunctions on motherhood and the outright condemnation of the practice of child marriage. Yet as Barbara Southard reminds us, the Bengali feminists in the nationalist period remained within the bounds of 'social feminism' that stopped short of demanding equality with men.[101] That also accounts for their ideological commitment towards upholding the nationalist perception of woman as mother and wife. No wonder, the conceptualisation of women in the wife–mother role remained largely unchallenged even by the most critical women writers of the period.

The incipient feminist consciousness that permeated the women's writings in the early twentieth century offers meaningful insights into the subtle shifts in the women's question that took place at the turn of the century. In a cultural ambience created by the Brahmo reformers from the mid-nineteenth century onwards that was particularly conducive to the education of women, the Wood's Despatch of 1854 played a significant role in triggering expansion of female school education in Bengal. From the 1880s, under the influence of Samadarshi Dal – a liberal group formed out of the Brahmo Samaj – college education (including medical education for women) expanded. By 1900, a substantial proportion of the middle-class women in Bengal, as compared to the Bombay and Madras Presidencies, had graduated from Calcutta University.[102]

In the first two decades of the twentieth century, participation of women in public sphere was facilitated by their employment as teachers and doctors.[103] In Bengal, the trend of women embracing career in medicine and later scientific education was shaped by the ideals of the later day Brahmo Samaj leaders. The Brahmo reformers worked towards promoting greater cooperation between men and women by, for instance, encouraging them to sit together in religious prayer meetings from the 1870s or welcoming bhadramahila in social gatherings such as tea parties.[104] Some of the later days Brahmo Samaj leaders such as Shibnath Sastri, Manmohan Ghose and Dwarkanath Ganguly, who went on to form the Sadharan Brahmo Samaj in 1878, fought against 'double standards in education for men and women'.[105] Dwarkanath Ganguly, for instance, encouraged science and medical education for women on the ground that women had right to similar kind of knowledge that was hitherto meant exclusively for men.[106] By the 1920s, awareness of the need for 'self-development' amongst literate bhadramahila had grown strong and the opportunity offered to them by Gandhi to participate in political activities led to an increased demand for higher education including science education as evident in the *Sixth Quinquennial Report on the Progress of Education in Bengal* (1917–18 and 1921–22).[107] Awareness of the ills of child marriage, early pregnancies, infant mortality and silent sufferings that often went undiagnosed earlier forced a critical evaluation of the oppressive social conditions under which they languished.[108]

Following bhadralok's deepening involvement in nationalist politics in the wake of the anti-partition agitation in 1905, educated women embraced the task of promoting their own cause. Women's question at the turn of the century essentially pivoted around educational reforms and eradication of certain social practices such as child marriage. The *mahila samitis* (women's organisation) such as the *Banga Mahila Samaj* (1879) and *Sakhi Samiti* (1886) which were founded by educated middle-class women from elite families promoted education and employment of widows, also holding discussions on subjects like science and hygiene and certain aspects of gender relationships.[109]

It was not before the Gandhian era of the 1920s that the political demands of women as right-bearing subjects began to be articulated on a national scale, indicating a major break from the nationalist patriarchal paradigm that had hitherto set the parameters of women's question.[110] In Bengal, as Barbara Southard's detailed study of women's movement from 1921 to 1936 suggests, the *Bangiya Nari Samaj* and the Bengali Women's Education League fought for women's suffrage and inclusion of girls in universal education schemes, respectively. Women's suffrage was, however, not perceived by the Bengali female activists as an isolated political issue but as a viable political weapon to promote social and educational reforms in favour of women.[111] The resolution of women's question no longer lay in reforming women but in uprooting certain societal practices, on behalf of women, the most telling example being the appeal of women to modify the institution of child marriage that eventually led to the passing of the Sarda Act in 1929.[112]

The booming print culture had already opened up new discursive spaces for literate women from the latter half of the nineteenth century. The writings of women authors like Krishnabhabini Das, Swarnakumari Devi and of numerous such contributors to women's journals in the late nineteenth century were charged with emancipatory potentials

that occasionally transcended the bounds of male-controlled intellectual discourse.[113] The demands for higher education, for instance,
were carefully laced with notions of personal and social advancement,
and as Krishnabhabini's writings revealed, a thrust towards 'economic
viability' and greater social power.[114]

However, child marriage and female education continued to remain
the two most relevant issues in the women's demands for social
and educational reforms, being discussed and debated persistently
from the second half of the nineteenth century. As early as in 1863,
Kailashbashini Devi noted in *Hindu Mahilaganer Hinabastha* (The
Woeful Plight of Hindu Women) the dangers of child marriage by
highlighting its relation to early maternity and its debilitating impact
on the health of the mother and the infant:

> Unless child marriage is prevented, our land will never have hap-
> piness and prosperity, marital harmony will never be established
> and girl children will never escape the harrowing torment of wid-
> owhood; child marriage has emerged as one of the main reasons
> for the backwardness of the Bengalis . . . there are instances of
> twelve or thirteen year old girls getting in the family way, thereby
> putting themselves in grave danger. Some leave this world along
> with the new-born . . . Some escape this fate themselves but lose
> their beloved infants . . . Maybe the new mother contracts post-
> natal maladies which cause extreme suffering; or else the infant is
> very sick and emaciated, adding to the parents' woes.[115]

At the turn of the century, educated middle-class women substantially absorbed the bhadralok concerns for the unhygienic nature of
midwifery practices in the *sutikagriha* and also the presumed dangers
of leaving the mother and the infant to the care of the uneducated
dhais. Women's writings in journals like *Antahpur* echoed such concerns and voiced the need for modernising birthing practices.[116] Such
writings should not, however, blind us to what the larger majority of
middle-class women might have desired in terms of medical attendance during childbirth. As Maneesha Lal reminds us the ordinary
middle-class women could have still continued to prefer hiring local
dhais who were easily accessible and affordable.[117]

However, women writers' views oscillated from being moderate
in seeking reform of their existing health conditions to being radical
in linking deteriorating health conditions to other societal maladies
that were alleged to have been perpetuated by the coercive patriarchal
structure in Bengal. Two essays that appeared in *Antahpur* in 1901

and 1903 poignantly captured the divergent positions held by women writers.

The first essay entitled *Bharat Mahilar Svasthya* ('Health of Indian Women') written by the editor of *Antahpur*, Hemantakumari Chaudhury, underscored the deplorable state of health of the *grihakatri* (mistress of the household) that provided the most powerful context for making health education an indispensable component of the curriculum for female education. A plea was, therefore, made for health education to be placed on the same plane as 'housecraft, child rearing and cooking'. In a lamenting note she stated:

> In recent times, women's education is progressing with great speed and every year, several girls after acquiring degrees from school are becoming famous. But probing into their health conditions reveals what? Most of them suffer from poor eyesight, mental ailments or other diseases. Violation of the principles of health is the main reason. These days, our attention is towards the outside world. Often, there are protest movements on whether roads are being kept clean under the supervision of the Municipalities. But nobody seems to have the time to think about the conditions of women in the antahpur. Has anyone who is born and reared in the antahpur and has inseparable and lasting ties with the space till death, ever reflected on the conditions of the women residing there? *It is despairing to see the ill-health of the mistress of the household on whom depends the peace and prosperity of the family, society and the nation.*(emphasis mine)[118]

This essay highlights the centrality of women's health in the progress of family, society and nation. Since the political contours of modern nation were yet to be outlined, nation here might have been used in a cultural sense to convey the idea of *Samaj* which, as Swarupa Gupta argues, was 'an-umbrella-like concept' that could encompass families, race, castes and religions and was a powerful conceptual category in forging Bengali identity and nationhood in the pre-modern era.[119] In driving home the importance of good physical health in enabling a woman to effectively perform household chores and responsibilities towards husband and children, the author explicitly conforms to the patriarchal position on what an ideal woman's role should be at home, in society and towards the nation. Yet, by pondering on the bodily ills plaguing the life of women, she hints at the poor status of women in Bengali society but quite evidently abstains from an outright criticism of patriarchy.

The publication of this essay evoked a riveting response from an ordinary housebound woman who chose to accord centrality to the uterus in explicating the various ills associated with the reproductive life of women. It is illustrative of how a section of the Bengali bhadramahila had shed their reticence by the turn of the century and broached the subject of their health in the public arena.[120]

The next essay entitled *Mahilar Svasthya* ('Women's Health') was written in 1903 by a woman writer who preferring anonymity called herself 'an ordinary Hindu woman'. This essay is perhaps more illuminating in terms of the manner in which it chose to explicate the decline in the physical, mental and reproductive health of women. In so doing, it transcended the restrictive boundaries of the patriarchal Bengali society and articulated an incipient but distinct feminist consciousness. It boldly interrogated those deeply entrenched social customs of child marriage and early motherhood that were sanctioned and seemingly normalised in the revivalist-patriarchal discourse of the late nineteenth century. It identified three reasons for the deterioration of health of Bengali women: bearing too many children at a young age, the moral degradation of men and, lastly, laziness of women. Instead of directly denouncing child marriage, early consummation was condemned as a potent evil affecting a young bride's health while early motherhood was squarely blamed for an entire range of sociocultural deprivations suffered by women. The essay stated:

> Young mothers not only are not able to entertain their husbands but are also incapable of showering the infant with affection . . . 90% of the middle-class women are deprived of proper nutrition and care . . . The concern of the husband's family is to see whether the daughter-in-law could give birth to an offspring but no one bothers about her health. Some women die immediately after giving birth. The rest keep conceiving every year. How can such *frequent pregnancies* ensure good health? Today, in the Hindu homes, the 16/17 year old girls are seen to be mother of three/four children . . . my dear sisters, *if we don't look after our body, who else will?*(emphasis mine)[121]

The subjectivity of the female writer is clearly evident in the audacious manner in which she chose to invoke the subject of moral depravity of men. A sorrowful picture is painted of the mental agony of the young mother who being burdened with the task of rearing so many children that left her tired and emaciated was forced to deprive her husband of adequate care and love. Such husbands looked for pleasure in the prostitutes' quarters. Ruminating on this moral degeneration the author of the essay finally wondered

> why so many young men in losing their moral character are also falling prey to new diseases and losing their lives? . . . even being alive so many of them are getting afflicted with obnoxious diseases that are jeopardising the lives of their wives and the future race. Why isn't anybody giving a thought to such evils?[122]

This article therefore constituted a powerful critique of patriarchy. It sought to establish women's control over their own bodies as simultaneously a liberating and empowering exercise. Yet what remained unaltered in these early expressions of feminism was the continued adherence to the cultural categories of *Janani* (motherhood) and *grihini* (mistress of the household) as the only valid frames of references in defining the essence of womanhood. Such cultural categories placed women, in their own perception, at the heart of the national agenda of progress and regeneration.

## Conclusion

Much of the western medical ideas on midwifery that were disseminated through the women's journals in the nineteenth century (such as debates on the need for hygienic *sutikaghar* or importance of the disproportion of the size of foetal head and pelvic structure in detecting abnormal birth or even the denunciation of dhais) acquired centrality in the nationalist discourse on maternal and child welfare in the twentieth century. In a significant way, therefore, nineteenth-century debates could be said to have laid the discursive groundwork for twentieth-century discourse on the subject. Only the context and the rationale had changed. While the nineteenth-century arguments were driven by reason and the bhadralok urge to modernise and self-improve, the twentieth-century ones had explicit nationalist and political overtones and often got drawn into a highly charged emotional debate on motherhood and future of the Bengali race.

To conclude, therefore, in the nineteenth century, modern scientific ideas of childbirth, child rearing and the general issue of women's health were gradually finding their way into the fabric of the Bengali society. Practices were slow to change. Yet there was an increasing awareness of the need to wrest midwifery from the control of the dhais and place it in the hands of trained professionals. The starting point was the incorporation of midwifery into the medical curriculum of

Calcutta University in 1841 followed by the rise of a class of male and female practitioners with their distinctive contributions to the field. To that we turn in the next chapter.

## Notes

1 W.R. Arney, *Power and the Profession of Obstetrics*, Chicago and London: Chicago University Press, 1982, 27.
2 Gyan Prakash, *Another Reason: Science and Imagination of Modern India*, Princeton, NJ: Princeton University Press, 1999; Dhruv Raina and S. Irfan Habib, *Domesticating Modern Science: A Social History of Science and Culture in Colonial India*, Tulika Books, New Delhi, 2004.
3 Partha Chatterjee, 'Our Modernity', in Partha Chatterjee, ed. *Empire and Nation: Selected Essays*, New York: Columbia University Press, 2010.
4 Samarpita Mitra, 'The Literary Public Sphere in Bengal: Aesthetics, Culture and Politics, 1905–1939', Unpublished PhD dissertation, University of Syracuse, 2009, 6l.
5 Of late, Samarpita Mitra has extensively studied the expansion of a literary sphere enabled by the booming print culture where a 'sub-national' and cultural identity of the Bengalis was worked out. The study has, however, excluded the health magazines from the scope of its enquiry, its focus being primarily on the formation of cultural identity and aesthetic sensibilities of the Bengalis in the nationalist period. For details, see Samarpita Mitra, 'The Literary Public Sphere'. The only scholar to have focused to some extent on the role of health journals in diffusing modern scientific ideas on health is Pradip Kumar Bose. See Pradip Kumar Bose, ed. *Health and Society in Bengal: A Selection from Late 19th-Century Bengali Periodicals*, New Delhi: Sage, 2006.
6 I have deliberately excluded the medical journals such as *Bishakdarpana* and *Anubikshan* from the scope of this chapter as they contained matters of academic interest and published with the aim of expanding professional knowledge in various branches of medicine. They were read by medical professionals and very rarely by non-medical lay public.
7 I have deliberately kept out the medical journals such as *Bishakdarpana* and *Anubikshan* from the scope of this chapter as they dealt more with diseases and their remedies than with the sociocultural ramifications of health problems in Bengal.
8 Geraldine Forbes, 'Education to Earn: Training Women in the Medical Professions', in Geraldine Forbes, ed. *Women in Colonial India: Essays on Politics, Medicine and Historiography*, New Delhi: Chronicle Books, 2005.
9 An essay on *Dhatribidya* (Midwifery) was translated from Dr James Simpson's lectures on the duties of a midwife during labour. Dr James Simpson rose to prominence in nineteenth-century England for his discovery of chloroform in 1847. For details, see Patricia Branca, *Silent Sisterhood: Middleclass Women in the Victorian Home*, London: Croom Helm, 1978, 84.
10 Gauri Viswanathan, *Masks of Conquest: Literary Study and British Rule in India*, New York: Columbia University Press, 1989, 146; John

McGuire, *The Making of a Colonial Mind: A Quantitative Study of the Bhadralok in Calcutta, 1857–1885*, Canberra: Australian National University, 1983; S.N. Mukherjee, 'The Bhadraloks of Bengal', in Dipankar Gupta, ed. *Social Stratification*, Delhi: Oxford University Press, 1991; B.B. Misra, *The Indian Middle Classes: Their Growth in Modern Times*, London, New York and Bombay: Oxford University Press, 1961, 10; By J.H. Broomfield's definition, the bhadralok were 'a socially privileged and consciously superior group, economic dependent upon landed rents and professional and clerical employment; keeping its distance from the masses by its acceptance of high caste proscriptions and its command of education'. J.H. Broomfield, *Elite Conflict in a Plural Society: Twentieth Century Bengal*, Berkeley and Los Angeles: University of California Press, 1968, 13.

11  Judith Walsh, 'The Virtuous Wife and the Well-Ordered Home: The Reconceptualisation of Bengali Women and Their Worlds', in Rajat Kanta Ray, ed. *Mind, Body and Society: Life and Mentality in Colonial Bengal*, Calcutta: Oxford University Press, 1995, 333.

12  Ashish Nandy, *The Intimate Enemy: Loss and Recovery of Self Under Colonialism*, Delhi: Oxford University Press, 1988.

13  Gauri Viswanathan, *Masks of Conquest: Literary Study and British Rule in India*, New York: Columbia University Press, 1989, 44, 146.

14  Ibid.

15  Ibid.

16  Sumit Sarkar, *Writing Social History*, New Delhi: Oxford University Press, 1997.

17  Tapan Raychaudhuri, 'The Pursuit of Reason in 19th-Century Bengal', in Rajat Kanta Ray, ed. *Mind, Body and Society: Life and Mentality in Colonial Bengal*, Calcutta: Oxford University Press, 1995, 48–52.

18  Prakash, *Another Reason*, 52.

19  Deepak Kumar, 'Calcutta: The Emergence of a Science City (1784–1856)', *Indian Journal of History of Science*, Vol.29, No.1, 1994, 1–7. Also see Srabani Sen, 'The Asiatic Society and the Sciences in India, 1784–1947', in Uma Dasgupta, ed. *Science and Modern India: An Institutional History, c.1784–1947*, New Delhi: Centre for Studies in Civilisations, 2011.

20  Prakash, *Another Reason*, 52.

21  Tanika Sarkar, 'Hindu Wife, Hindu Nation: Domesticity and Nationalism in Nineteenth-Century Bengal', in Tanika Sarkar, ed. *Hindu Wife, Hindu Nation: Community, Religion, and Cultural Nationalism*, New Delhi: Permanent Black, 2001, 31–37.

22  Mrinalini Sinha, *Colonial Masculinity: The 'Manly Englishman' and the 'Effeminate Bengali' in the Late 19th Century*, Manchester and New York: Manchester University Press, 1995.

23  John Rosselli, 'The Self-Image of Effeteness: Physical Education and Nationalism in 19th Century Bengal', *Past and Present*, Vol. 86, 1980, 121–148.

24  'The Revival of National Physical Health', *Cikitsa Sammilani,* April–May, 1885 quoted in Pradip Bose, *Health and Society*, 105.

25  Ibid., 108.

26  Mel Gorman, 'Introduction of Western Science into Colonial India: Role of the CMC', *Proceedings of the American Philosophical Society*, Vol.128, No.2, 1988, 276–298.

27  Christian Hochmuth, 'Patterns of Medical Culture in Colonial Bengal, 1835–1880', *Bulletin of the History of Medicine*, Vol.80, No.1, 2006, 39–72.

28  David Arnold, 'Medical Priorities and Practice in 19th British India', *South Asia Research*, Vol.5, No.2, 1985, 167–183; Prakash, *Another Reason*.

29  'The Revival of National Physical Health', 105.

30  Projit Bihari Mukharji, *Nationalising the Body: Medical Market, Print and Daktari Medicine*, London: Anthem Press, 2011.

31  Gourinath Sengupta, *Sharirik Svasthya Bidhan* (A Treatise on Physical Health), Calcutta: 1862, Introduction.

32  Sengupta, *Sharirik Svasthya Bidhan*.

33  '*Svasthyaraksha: Griha Parishkar (Preserving Health: Cleaning the House)*', *Bamabodhini Patrika*, Vol.1, No.1, 1864, 11–12. This essay prescribed ways to keep the house clean. The second essay in the series provided instructions on how to keep clothes clean. See '*Svasthyaraksh: Bastra Parishkar*' (*Preserving Health: Cleaning the Clothes*), *Bamabodhini Patrika*, Vol.1, No.5, December 1864, 79–80. The third essay prescribed ways to keep the body clean. See '*Svasthyaraksha: Deha Parishkar*', *Bamabodhini Patrika*, Vol.1, No.7, 1865, 77–80.

34  '*Sharirik Svasthyabidhan*', *Bamabodhini Patrika*, Vol.3, No.52, Nov.1867, 640–642. It was only a part of such series of essays published in 1867 and 1868.

35  Jordanova has alluded to the inclination of men in eighteenth-century France and England to supervise women in childbirth without getting directly involved in it. The same process could be seen to be at work in nineteenth-century Bengal. Bengali bhadraloks were seen to advise women on everything from running a household to giving birth. For details see L.J. Jordanova, 'Natural Facts: A Historical Perspective on Science and Sexuality', in Carol P. MacCormack and Marilyn Strathern, eds. *Nature, Culture and Gender*, Cambridge: Cambridge University Press, 1980.

36  Amiya P. Sen, *Hindu Revivalism in Bengal, 1872–1905: Some Essays in Interpretation*, Delhi: Oxford University Press, 1993.

37  Tanika Sarkar, 'Conjugality and Hindu Nationalism: Resisting Colonial Reason and the Death of a Child-Wife', in Tanika Sarkar, ed. *Hindu Wife, Hindu Nation*, 196–197. The discriminatory policies included the repressive vernacular press acts of the 1870s issued by Viceroy Lytton, and the staunch opposition of the British to the Ilbert Bill introduced by Viceroy Ripon in 1883 that allowed British offenders to be tried by Indian Judges and Magistrates. The protests launched by the British in India and Britain brought to the fore the racist nature of the colonial rule in India.

38  Haranath Ray's book received positive reviews at that time from contemporary newspapers such as *Indian Daily News*, *The Statesman*, *Indian Mirror*, *the Hope*, *Bangabashi*, *Sanjivani* and *the Amrita Bazar Patrika*. The book was considered to be useful not only to the medical practitioners but also to the ordinary people living in the 'remotest corner of the interior'. See 'Advertisement: Dhatree-Siksha by Babu Haronath Roy, LMS', *The Amrita Bazar Patrika*, 24 November 1887.

39  Haranath Ray, *Dhatri-Sikkha Samgraha* (Midwife's Vade-Mecum), Calcutta: Bengal Law Report Press, 1887, 349–359.

40 In a slightly different context, Mark Singleton has remarkably showed how Indian yogic practices at the turn of the century incorporated and 'indigenised' certain aspects of the late nineteenth-century social ideologies of social Darwinism and eugenics in an attempt to 'recast modern science as ancient truth'. Mark Singleton, 'Yoga, Eugenics and Spiritual Darwinism in the Early Twentieth Century', *International Journal of Hindu Studies*, Vol.11, No.2, 2007, 138.

41 Sarkar, 'Conjugality and Hindu Nationalism', 197.

42 Sinha, *Colonial Masculinity*, Chapter 4.

43 Charles Heimsath, 'The Origin and Enactment of the Indian Age of Consent Bill, 1891', *The Journal of Asian Studies*, Vol.21, No.4, 1962, 491–504.

44 Sen, *Hindu Revivalism in Bengal*, 379.

45 Ibid., 392.

46 See for instance, 'The Age of Consent Bill', *Dainik o Samacara Chandrika*, 25 January 1891, R.N.P (Reports on Native Newspapers); Boyle Chunder Sen, 'The Calcutta Medical Society: The Nubile Age of Females in India', *Indian Medical Gazette*, Vol.25, 1890, 306–312.

47 Judith Walsh, 'The Virtuous Wife'. Meredith Borthwick has analysed the reconstitution of domesticity, conjugality and motherhood in colonial Bengal between 1849 and 1905. For details see Meredith Borthwick, *The Changing Role of Women in Bengal, 1849–1905*, Princeton, NJ: Princeton University Press, 1984, Chapters 4, 5 and 6.

48 Kumar Harendra Krishna was the Maharaj (King) of Hathwah and one who received the title of 'Bahadur' for his loyalty to the government. He also served as the vice-president of the Asiatic Society in 1868.

49 Kumar Harendra Krishna, *A Lecture on Female Education in Bengal: Delivered at the Bethune Society*, Calcutta: Bengalee Press, 1863.

50 Borthwick, *The Changing Role of Women*, Chapter 3; Malavika Karlekar 'Kadambini and the Bhadralok: Early Debates Over Women's Education in Bengal', *Economic and Political Weekly*, Vol.21, No.19, 1986, 25–31.

51 Krishna Sen, 'Lessons in Self-Fashioning: "Bamabodhini Patrika" and the Education of Women in Colonial Bengal', *Victorian Periodicals Review*, Vol.37, No.2, 2004, 177.

52 Some of the essays on women's education on health, literature, science, geography, etc. which were published in *Bamabodhini Patrika* were later compiled in the form of a book named as *Narisiksa* ('Female Education') and published under the auspices of the *Bamabodhini Sabha*. The book was praised in press as a remarkable contribution to the advancement of female education. See Bharati Ray, *Shekaler Nari Siksha: Bamabodhini Patrika (1270–1399)*, Calcutta: Women's Studies Research Centre, 1998, 71–75.

53 'Ramanir Kartabya,' *Bamabodhini Patrika*, February 1887, No.265, 302–306.

54 It falls in line with L.J. Jordanova's compelling argument about how the identification of women with 'nature' and men with 'culture' in eighteenth-century England and France was being garbed in a scientific and medical language and, hence, served to justify and naturalise the control of men as forces of modernity, enlightenment and progress over women as irrational, superstitious and traditional. Jordanova, 'Natural Facts'.

55  Karlekar, 'Kadambini and the Bhadralok'.
56  '*Ramanir Kartabya* (Duties of a Woman)', *Bamabodhini Patrika*, Vol.3, No.262, December 1886, 230–231. Similar views were expressed in another prominent but women-run magazine entitled *Antahpur* at the turn of the century. See for instance, '*Grihaswasthye Ramanir Drishti* (Attention of Women towards Household Chores)', *Antahpur*, Vol.VII, No.IX, January 1905, 210–213.
57  See David Arnold and Sumit Sarkar, 'In Search of Rational Remedies: Homeopathy in 19th-Century Bengal', in Waltraud Ernst, ed. *Plural Medicine: Tradition and Modernity, 1800–2000*, London and New York: Routledge, 2000, 40–57. Also see Das, 'Debating Scientific Medicine'.
58  '*Garhasthya Cikitsa Pranali* (Methods of Home Treatment)', *Bamabodhini Patrika*, Vol.8, No.100, December 1871, 242.
59  '*Svasthya Raksha*', *Bangamahila*, Vol.1, No.5, 1875. Similar essays were published in other contemporary journals. For instance, see '*Svasthyaraksha o Shorir Palan* (Preservation and Care of Health)', *Paricarika*, Vol.4, No.2, July 1882, 24–27.
60  Shib Chunder Bose, *Sisupalan*, Part I, Serampore: Mission Press, 1857, Introduction.
61  See '*Dhatribidya: Sutikagar* (The art of Midwifery: The Site of Birth)', *Bamabodhini Patrika*, Vol.3, No.52, November 1867, 636. Concerns for child mortality continued to be expressed as a sign of unscientific ways of conducting birth in Bengali households. See, for example, '*Svasthya*', *Bharati*, Vol.1, No.5, 1877, 180–183; Nanibala Dasi, '*Sutikagar e prasutir Cikitsa* (Care of Pregnant Woman at the Site of Birth)', *Antahpur*, Vol.6, No.5, August 1903.
62  'Scraps and Comments', *The Amrita Bazar Patrika*, 19 October 1876.
63  Hemantakumari Chaudhury, '*Sutikagriha* (The Site of Birth)', *Antahpur*, Vol.9, 1902, 133.
64  J.A. Bourdillon, *Report of the Census of Bengal, 1881*, Vol.1, Calcutta: Bengal Secretariat Press, 1883, 68. Earlier one official report of 1873 concluded that mortality amongst 'infants and young children' was higher in Bengal than in England and any lower figure of infant mortality that might have been published in the previous returns was solely due to 'deficient registration'. See *Ordinary General Mortality in the Districts in Bengal, Including the Mortality in Selected Areas*, Part I, 1873, 7.
65  A series on the symptoms and treatment of neonatal tetanus was published in *Cikista Sammilani* in 1886 according to allopathy, homeopathy and Ayurveda. See Jagabandhu Basu, '*Allopathy: Anture Chheler PechoyePawa Rog* (Neonatal Tetanus of the Infant)', *Cikitsa Sammilani*, Vol.2, 1886, 180–182, 216–218; Annadacharan Khastagir, '*Homeopathy: Nabaprasuto Sisur Dhanushtankar Rog* (Neonatal Tetanus of the New-Born Infant)', *Cikitsa Sammilani*, Vol.2, 1886, 218–220; Abinashchandra Kaviratna, '*Baidyamate Anturchheler Rog* (Neonatal Tetanus of Infant according to Ayurveda)', 183–185 and 220–224.
66  The subscription list of *Cikitsa Sammilani* shows a large number of non-medical people as regularly subscribing and reading the journal. They included deputy magistrates in the districts, zamindars, 'head clerks', lawyers of High Court Calcutta and 'head pundits' who were possibly teachers. See, for instance, '*Mulyaprapti* (Subscription List)', *Cikitsa Sammilani*,

Vol.3, 1887 and '*Mulyaprapti* (Subscription List)', *Cikitsa Sammilani*, Vol.4, 1884.

67 Margaret Ida Balfour and Ruth Young, *The Work of Medical Women in India*, Oxford: Oxford University Press, 1929, 81. David Arnold has acknowledged the overall role of missionaries in penetrating the 'uncolonised' space of zenana. See Arnold, *Colonising the Body*, 256.

68 In as early as 1848, the annual report of the newly opened midwifery ward of the CMC declared with pride that six of their college graduates had successfully settled in and around Calcutta and were managing labour cases of women although that mostly excluded direct manual interference with their body parts. It also stated that the practice of confining women to sutikaghar/anturghar was 'entirely abandoned by all the respectable natives in Calcutta'. Meredith Borthwick in her extensive study of the bhadramahila has considered this statement to be 'far too sweeping expression of optimism'. See Borthwick, *Changing Role of Women*, 156–157.

69 West Bengal State Archives (WBSA), Proceedings of the Lieutenant Governor of Bengal, General Department, Medical Branch, Progs No.1–7, August 1867. However, the CMC had begun to teach midwifery from 1841 along with surgery, botany and medical jurisprudence. See CMC, Centenary Volume, Calcutta: Statesman Press, 1935. This incident has been discussed in greater detail in Chapter 2.

70 Krishna Sen states that every copy of the magazine was sold out till similar magazines began to appear in the last quarter of the nineteenth century. Sen, 'Lessons in Self-Fashioning', 177.

71 '*Dhatribidya* (Midwifery)', *Bamabodhini Patrika*, Vol.3, No.50, September 1867, 597.

72 '*Dhatribidya: Garbhabasthyay Prasutir Susrusa* (Care of Pregnant Women)', *Bamabodhini Patrika*, Vol.3, No.51, November 1867, 616–619.

73 '*Dhatribidya: Sutikagar* (The Site of Birth),' *Bamabodhini Patrika*, Vol.3, No.52, November–December 1867, 636–637.

74 '*Dhatribidya: Swabhabik Prasab* (Normal Labour)', *Bamabodhini Patrika*, Vol.3, No.53, December 1867, 656.

75 '*Dhatribidya: Dhatrir Kartabya* (Duties of a Midwife)', *Bamabodhini Patrika*, Vol.3, No.54, January 1868, 676.

76 '*Dhatribidya: Dhatrir Kartabya* (Duties of a Midwife)'.

77 Hendrik Van Deventer, a renowned Dutch obstetrician, mentioned the disproportion between the size of the pelvis and the head of the foetus in his eighteenth-century work on midwifery. For details see Jean Donnison, *Midwives and Medical Men: A History of the Struggle for the Control of Childbirth*, London: Historical Publications Ltd, 1993.

78 '*Svasthya*', *Bharat*, Vol.1, No.5, 1877, 180–183.

79 '*Matrigarbha o Garbhasisu* (Mother's Womb and the Foetus Within)', *Bamabodhini Patrika*, Vol.8, No.109, September 1872.

80 '*Svasthya*', *Bharati*.

81 How many dhais availed of those books is not known. But it was assumed that the lucidity of the Bengali language could help the dhais in grasping the information contained in such pamphlets.

82 Jadunath Mukhopadhyaya, *Dhatrisiksha ebong prasutisiksha arthat kathopakathanchhale dhai ebong Prasutidiger proti upadesh* (Educating

the Midwife and the Pregnant Woman Written in the Form of Dialogue), Chinsurah: Chikitsabodak Press, 1867.

83 Annada Charan Khastagir, *Manabjanmatattva, Dhatribidya, Nabaprasut Sisu o Strijatir Byadhisangraha* (A Treatise on the Science and Practice of Midwifery with Diseases of Children and Women), Second Edition, Calcutta: Girish Vidyaratna, 1878.

84 Khirodaprosad Chattopadhyay, *Dhatribidya* (Midwifery), Bhowanipur: Oriental Press, 1886.

85 One Kumudini Sinha raised her children following the guidelines in Annada Charan Khastagir's treatise. This has been mentioned by Meredith Borthwick. See Borthwick, *The Changing Role of Women*, 163.

86 Shib Chunder Deb, *Sisupalan*, Part II, Calcutta, 1868.

87 Borthwick, *Changing Role of Women*, Chapter 5. Also see Branca, *Silent Sisterhood*, Chapter six.

88 A series of articles entitled '*Sisu Palan* (Infant Rearing)' was published in all the issues of *Bamabodhini Patrika* in 1868 and 1869. See 'Sisu Palan' *Bamabodhini Patrika*, Vol.4, 1868 and Vol.5, 1869.

89 Iqbal Singh Sevea, *The Political Philosophy of Muhammad Iqbal: Islam and Nationalism in Late Colonial India*, New York: Cambridge University Press, 2012, 69–70.

90 Sonia Nishat Amin, *The World of Muslim Women in Colonial Bengal, 1876–1939*, Leiden, New York and Koln: E.J. Brill, 1996, 93–96.

91 Karlekar, 'Kadambini and the Bhadralok'.

92 WBSA, Judicial Department (Medical Branch), File No.63, Progs No:7–9, December 1873.

93 Sean Lang, 'Saving India Through Its Women', *History Today*, Vol.55, No.9, 2009, 46–47.

94 The aversion of middle-class Bengali women of the zenana to seeking medical aid from a male doctor turned out to be one of the chief motivating forces for the institutionalisation of women's medicine and professionalisation of women doctors in Victorian Britain. See Antoinette Burton, 'Contesting the *Zenana*: The Mission to Make Lady Doctors for India, 1874–1885', *The Journal of British Studies*, Vol.35, No.3, 1996, 368–398.

95 Balfour and Young, *The Work of Medical Women*, 20–21. For a general outline of the Dufferin Fund, see Arnold, *Colonising the Body*, 260–268; Maneesha Lal, 'The Politics of Gender and Medicine in Colonial India: The Countess of Dufferin Fund, 1885–1888', *Bulletin of the History of Medicine*, Vol.68, No.1, Spring 1994, 29–66.

96 Supriya Guha, 'From Dais to Doctors: The Medicalisation of Childbirth in Colonial India', in Lakhsmi Lingam, ed. *Understanding Women's Health Issues: A Reader*, New Delhi: Kali, 1998, 145–162.

97 Supriya Guha, ' "The Best Swadeshi": Reproductive Health in Bengal, 1840–1940', in Sarah Hodges, ed. *Reproductive Health in India: History, Politics, Controversies*, Delhi: Orient Longman, 2006.

98 Ghulam Murshid, *Reluctant Debutante: Response of Bengali Women to Modernisation, 1849–1905*, Rajshahi: Sahitya Samsad, 1985, See Introduction and Chapter 3.

99 Himani Bannerji, 'Fashioning a Self: Educational Proposals for and by Women in Popular Magazines in Colonial Bengal', *Economic and Political Weekly*, Vol.26, No.43, 1991, 50.

100 Anindita Ghosh, *Behind the Veil: Resistance, Women and the Everyday in Colonial South Asia*, Delhi: Permanent Black, 2007. This point is made by Ghosh drawing upon similar arguments made earlier by Ranajit Guha in 'The Career of an Anti-God in Heaven and on Earth', in Asok Mitra, ed. *The Truth Unites*, Calcutta: Subarnarekha, 1985.

101 Barbara Southard, *The Women's Movement and Colonial Politics in Bengal: The Quest for Political Rights, Education and Social Reform Legislation, 1921–1936*, New Delhi: Mahohar, 1995, Chapter 3.

102 For instance, the reports on the Progress of Education in India for the year 1902 show that in that year, out of the 177 female college students in India, 55 were from Bengal, with only 5 from Madras and 2 from Bombay and United Provinces. From 1897 to 1902, 37 women graduated from the Calcutta University as against 7 students from Madras, 1 from the United Province and 1 from Bombay. 'Progress of Education in India, 1897–1902', 299, quoted in Karlekar, 'Kadambini and the Bhadralok,' 29 and fn34. According to the Census of Calcutta, in 1901, literate women formed 9.7 per cent of the total female population as compared with 3.36 per cent in 1876. See Censuses for Calcutta, Towns and Suburbs, 1876, 1901 as quoted in Borthwick, *The Changing Role of Women*, fn181.

103 It was only after the Second World War that middle-class women took up jobs as stenographers, telephone operators, office girls etc. See Bharati Ray, 'Women of Bengal: Transformation in Ideas and Ideals, 1900–1947', *Social Scientist*, Vol.19, Nos.5–6, 1991, 11.

104 See Borthwick, *The Changing Role of Women*, 259–260.

105 See David Kopf, *Brahmo Samaj and the Shaping of Modern Mind*, Princeton, NJ: Princeton University Press, 1979, 124.

106 Karlekar, 'Kadambini and the Bhadralok', 26.

107 Rachana Chakraborty, 'Women's Education and Empowerment in Colonial Bengal', in Hans Hagerdal, ed. *Responding to the West: Essays on Colonial Agency and Asian Agency*, Amsterdam: Amsterdam University Press, 2009, 96.

108 Hemantakumari Chaudhury, 'Bharat Mahilar Svasthya (Health of Indian Women)', *Antahpur*, Vol.4, No.7, July 1901, 149–151.

109 Murshid, *Reluctant Debutante*, 94–95.

110 Ibid.

111 Southard, *The Women's Movement and Colonial Politics in Bengal*, Chapter 3.

112 Sinha, *Specters of Mother India*, 51.

113 Malini Bhattacharya has argued how education had the potential of empowering women although that power was used 'not merely to serve the revised needs of the family and the home, but for self-development and expression; it is a conceptual tool which allow the woman to critique effectively the various inequities of her social condition'. For details see Malini Bhattacharya and Abhijit Sen, eds. *Talking of Power: Early Writings of Bengali Women from the Mid-19th to the Beginning of the Twentieth Century*, Kolkata: Stree, 2003, 3.

114 Banerji, 'Fashioning a Self', 55–58.

115 Kailashbasini Devi, 'The Woeful Plight of Hindu Women', in Bhattacharya and Sen, ed. *Talking of Power*, 40.

116 See for instance, Dasi, 'Sutikagar e prasutir cikitsa'; Chaudhury, 'Sutikagriha'.
117 Lal, 'The Politics of Gender and Medicine'. Women like Kailashbashini Devi, Sudha Majumdar described their dhais as friendly and cooperative. See Chandrika Paul, 'The Uneasy Alliance: The Work of British and Bengali Medical Professionals, 1870–1935', Unpublished PhD dissertation, University of Cincinnati, 1997, 182–184.
118 Chaudhury, 'Bharat Mahilar Svasthya', 150.
119 Swarupa Gupta, 'Notions of Nationhood in Bengal: Perspectives on Samaj, 1867–1905', *Modern Asian Studies*, Vol.40, No.2, 2006, 273–302.
120 Sarojini Devi, 'Mahilar Svasthya Sambandhe Koyekti Katha (Few Words About Indian Women's Health)', *Antahpur*, Vol.4, No.12, December 1901, 269.
121 'Mahilar Svasthya (Women's Health)', *Antahpur*, Vol.4, No.3, June–July 1903, 58.
122 Ibid.

# 2 The art and science of midwifery

## Institutionalisation of midwifery and the constitution of a medical discourse, 1860s–1930s

In an introductory lecture on obstetrics to the students of Queen's College, Galway (Queen's University of Ireland) in 1878, Dr R. J. Kinkead alluded to midwifery and diseases of women as 'obstetrics' and 'gynaecology'. Underscoring the importance of obstetrics in medical science, Kinkead stated

> the fact is becoming more and more realised that obstetrics and gynaecology are portions of medical science requiring the highest faculties of mind to comprehend, containing problems the most intricate to solve, operations calling forth the most finished surgical skill, and affording a key to the study of general disease found in no other branch . . . there is no branch of your profession so important for you to know thoroughly as that relating to obstetrics and diseases of women.[1]

Kinkead's words point to a perceptible shift in the British medical profession's view of midwifery in the late nineteenth century.[2] By then, the medical profession had gradually ceased to consider it as a subject unworthy of being studied by a 'cultivated mind' or a 'powerful intellect'.[3] The earlier trend of depriving the practitioners of midwifery from fellowship of the College of Physicians and barring them from sitting in the council of the College of Surgeons prior to 1828 had also ceased. The promulgation of the Medical Amendment Act of 1886 further stipulated that examination in midwifery be made compulsory along with medicine and surgery for the purpose of registration of all practitioners.[4] The Act constituted a vital step towards making midwifery part of medical education and training in Britain. How much of the vision for improving medical education in obstetrics and gynaecology such as that underscored by Kinkead was appropriated and accommodated in the expanding western medical pedagogy in colonial Bengal?

Bengal being one of the strongholds of the British colonial empire in India fostered the most elaborate and well-entrenched medical establishment along western medical lines. Following the foundation of the Calcutta Medical College (CMC) in 1835, midwifery was incorporated into the syllabus of the College in 1841. The central concern of this chapter is to analyse the various axes around which medical education and practice of midwifery were instituted. The training of dhais or their replacement with midwives trained in western medicine constituted a principal axis. The other major axis, which also forms the key focus of the chapter, was the realignment of professional relationships between the female and male medical practitioners of midwifery, with the former dominating the realm of actual practice (i.e. attending women in childbirth) and the latter contributing to the more theoretical domain of midwifery education and research on obstetrics. The analytical framework of this chapter is shaped by the interrogation of the two streams of thought dominating the historiography of childbirth in the West and in India. In the West the incursion of surgery/technology into the realm of midwifery is unequivocally identified as an undisputed sign of male ascendancy in the profession. This line of interpretation perceived the displacement of female birth assistants by male physicians as the principal factor driving medicalisation and technological expansion of midwifery.[5] In contrast to western historiography, scholars in India cite the practice of seclusion amongst respectable Indian females as a powerful cultural constraint that, in their opinion, curbed male professional presence in midwifery and, hence, accounted for the centrality of the female doctors in medicalising childbirth in India.[6]

The chapter argues that in the case of Bengal medical intervention in childbirth did not reflect a clear-cut ascendancy of male medical professionals by marginalising/uprooting the dhais, as it was claimed to have happened in the West. Similarly, putting the sole spotlight on the agency of female medical practitioners in medicalising childbirth, as is the reigning tendency in Indian historiography, is also a classic instance of historical oversight. To address the lacuna, the chapter analyses the role of both female and male practitioners in marking their own spheres of dominance in the domain of midwifery. It brings into sharper historical focus the contribution of male physicians arguing that their role was more ideological and pedagogic, than being directly interventionist; it should not solely be understood through the constricted prism of professionalism but placed in a broader and more pervasive framework of nationalism. Medicalisation of childbirth, the chapter argues, was preceded by the constitution of a medical discourse on midwifery that led to it being redefined as the science of obstetrics, a process enabled by the incorporation of midwifery in the Calcutta University curriculum in the mid-nineteenth century under the supervision of the faculty of the CMC, consisting entirely of male doctors, both indigenous and British. Yet, the actual practice of midwifery as a specialised branch of medical science gained widespread acceptance with the intervention of female medical professionals as opposed to the lay midwives in the late nineteenth and early twentieth centuries.

## The art of midwifery

Prior to the ascendancy of the modern medical profession, midwifery was almost universally a female-regulated cultural domain, albeit structured around varied and region-specific ritualistic mores. The objective of this chapter is also to identify those sociocultural stereotypes that influenced the reconceptualisation of midwifery as a scientific–medical discipline and significantly affected its institutionalisation in colonial Bengal.

One of the earliest and professedly 'simple but faithful delineation' of Hindu social and cultural life with all its 'many incrusted defects and deficiencies still lurking in our social system' came from the pen of Shib Chunder Bose. As an 'enlightened' Brahmo and also having 'received the stirring impulse of western culture and thought', Bose claimed to produce a critical insider's account of the Hindu society in the late nineteenth century, which was chiefly intended for 'English readers' and for those engaged in the work of 'religious regeneration and social reform in India'.[7] Bose's critical description of the process of childbirth in a typical Hindu home in Bengal assumes greater significance in revealing the self-critical and deeply introspective mood of the western-educated Bengali middle class in the late nineteenth century.[8] To quote Bose,

> When the period of delivery arrives, and to her it is an awful period which can be more easily conceived than described, the girl writhing under agony is taken into a room called Sootikaghur or Antoorghur, where no male members of the family are admitted. She is made to wear a red-bordered robe and two images of the goddess Shashthi made of cow dung are placed near the threshold of the room for her daily worship . . . for one month – the period

of her confinement. If in her tender age, the labour be a protracted one, she often suffers greatly from the want of a skilful surgeon or even a proper midwife. Before the founding of that noble institution, the CMC, proper midwives were not available, because they had no systematic training; their profession was chiefly confined to the Dome and Bagthee caste.[9]

As Bose's account reveals, the whole gamut of practices regulating childbirth in early colonial Bengal was determined by age-old religious and cultural practices. Even the choice of the smallest and allegedly the most ill-ventilated room as the *sutikaghar* (where birth took place) was dictated by the imperative of keeping out 'demons' and 'malign spirits' and, more significantly, of shutting out the 'polluting' act of birth from the main premises of the household. The perception of the polluting nature of birth in Hindu ritual practices led to it being conducted by dhais belonging mostly to low, 'untouchable' castes such as Dome and Bagdi.

Cultural observances blending with popular cult worship continued well into the postnatal period. As Bose describes, this included the well-established and ubiquitous custom of invoking and worshipping goddess *Shashthi* as the 'protectress of children' on the sixth day after birth and performing the ceremony of *autcowroy* (eight cowries) on the eighth day. However, more rational and less rigorous alternatives to such time-honoured practices were also sometimes resorted to. One such variant was the *Hariloot* system in which the pregnant woman was spared of an array of strict observances followed in the older system such as abstaining from cold water or drinks and *jhal* (spices) and *thaap* (fire) after delivery. Under the modified Hariloot system, the length of seclusion from main household in the post-partum period was cut short from one month to one week by bathing the mother in cold water immediately after delivery and feeding her ordinary food of *dal vaath* (rice and lentils), curry, fish and tamarind.[10]

For the larger part of the nineteenth century, therefore, the process of childbirth remained firmly ensconced in a complex set of cultural and ritualistic practices controlled by the dhai and the female members of the household. As reverend Lal Behary Dey described in his portrayal of rural Bengal, the dhai/midwife being a key figure in the socio-cultural functions revolving around the occasion of birth was usually looked upon as a familiar, motherly figure having secret liaison with God (*Vidhata*) who confirmed the destiny of the child on the sixth night of birth.[11] Her remuneration varied according to the financial status of the family and the sex of the child, the delivery of a male child assuring greater sum of money and gifts. Moreover, her role was conceived more in social than in medical terms. It often stretched to include looking after the mother and her newborn child and performing few household chores, a trend that was evident in other parts of the world as well.

In the perception of the British medical professionals and missionaries, what set India apart from other countries in terms of response to western medical practice was the popular image of Indian women's abhorrence for instruments and operations. Such presumptions loomed large in official correspondence including the earlier annual reports of the Bengal Branch of the Dufferin Fund.[12] In some instances, women's fear of instruments was projected as being symptomatic of the strong aversion of the 'simple and timid' Indians, in general, towards surgery.[13] As late as in 1915, a missionary nurse from New Zealand who served in one of the outlying districts of India described the horrified reaction of two female relatives of a woman in labour on seeing instrument being introduced by the doctor, in the following words:

> When one of them sees instruments being introduced, she rushes yelling from the room and tells some awful tale to all those sitting outside. For a few minutes, it sounds as if there is going to be a riot: but we continue working and perspiring.[14]

The Indian women's aversion for instruments was, however, of marginal importance in colonial imagination when compared to the ubiquitousness of the image of Indian women trapped in the custom of seclusion (purdah). Purdah, it was assumed, impinged on the women's autonomy and their ability to seek professional medical help beyond the restrictive boundaries of home. The impenetrability of zenana emerged as a vital concern in the writings of contemporary medical practitioners, being perceived, for a long time, as a serious impediment to the institutionalisation of midwifery practice. According to such writings, well-entrenched notions of modesty and shame (*lajja*) that governed the cultural deportment of purdahnashin women dissuaded them from seeking medical assistance from a male doctor. For instance, Dr Margaret Balfour, one of the leading female practitioners in early twentieth-century India, stated in her account that 'it is in childbirth that the full horror of the purdah system is seen, when women are allowed to die undelivered sooner than show themselves to a man'.[15] Purdah system also accounted for the exclusion of midwifery from the syllabus of the Medical College before 1841 on the ground that 'from the peculiar customs and prejudices of the country, (midwifery) is an unnecessary accomplishment to the native practitioner'.[16] Maneesha Lal has aptly argued that purdah was overemphasised by the proponents of female medical aid who conveniently overlooked other major factors such as poverty, education, sanitation and nutrition as being equally responsible for limiting women's access to health care.[17]

It is interesting to note that midwifery was incorporated into the medical curriculum of the Calcutta University in 1841 amidst such perceived sociocultural constraints. Although that did not immediately alter the meaning of birth as practised by the Bengali dhais, the inclusion of midwifery as part of medical education did underscore the broadening of its epistemological dimensions and subsequent recasting as a scientific paradigm. It also marked the beginning of a long drawn-out process of its reconstitution under the professional and academic expertise of the medical faculty in Bengal, consisting largely of the Indian Medical Service (IMS) officials.

## The science of midwifery

The story of scientification of midwifery in Bengal is deeply associated with the inauguration of the CMC in 1835. The Medical College which institutionalised western medical science in India played a pivotal role in laying the basis of a new pedagogy on midwifery. The doctors of the IMS serving as professors in various branches of medicine provided the initial blueprint on which the teaching and training in midwifery were instituted. Yet the debates at the time of the foundation of the Medical College curiously point towards the initial reluctance of the colonial medical personnel towards establishing a lying-in hospital within the precinct of the college.

On being questioned about the utility of a scheme to establish a lying-in hospital by the Fever Hospital and Municipal Improvement Committee in 1838, Dr Madhusudhan Gupta expressed his deep-seated apprehensions.[18] Gupta strongly felt that 'owing to many insurmountable prejudices that prevail among all classes of the Natives, as to staying in Hospital', the utility of such a hospital would eventually be confined to the 'lower classes of the Natives' and the poor Muslim and Christian women.[19] Instead he proposed the creation of a lying-in ward with twenty beds to be attached to the newly established Fever Hospital and also encouraged the establishment of a 'school of midwifery'. The proposed school would be charged with the crucial tasks of delivering practical instructions on the anatomical details of pelvis and other vital reproductive organs to local women (and not those male students who were going into medical training) who would be trained as midwives for two years and awarded 'certificates of proficiency' on performing satisfactorily in the examinations. Thus, despite initial doubts, Gupta had at an early phase of the institutionalisation of western medicine envisioned the systematisation and rationalisation of midwifery practice in Bengal through training and education of indigenous females.[20]

In the midst of such profound misgivings, a lying-in hospital, with provision for the treatment of 100 women, was established in the Medical College in 1840. It was built with funds raised by public subscription. Its significance in instructing college students and in educating both European and 'native' midwives was emphasised in official correspondence as was the humanitarian concern of the colonial state for the 'loss of life' due to 'bad practice'.[21] Thus, the Governor General in Council assigned a sum of Rs 500 for expenses pertaining to the functioning of the hospital. Midwifery was introduced as a subject into the syllabus of the Medical College in 1841.

In 1849 separate professorships of anatomy and midwifery were established on a permanent basis. Mel Gorman highlights the centrality of clinical-anatomy in claiming the superiority of modern scientific medicine and in placing the Medical College at the 'top rank of teaching anatomy in the world'.[22] The separation of the chairs of anatomy and midwifery was therefore integral to any such scheme for further specialisation in different branches of modern medicine that included anatomy, physiology and pathology. In view of the 'increasing reputation of the college and its recognition by various medical bodies in this country', the financial department of the government consented to the permanent dissociation of the department of anatomy from that of midwifery. Thereupon, Assistant Surgeon W. Walker was appointed as the Professor of Anatomy while Dr Goodeve was reinstated as only the Professor of Midwifery that relieved him from his previous cumbrous role as the Professor of Anatomy and Midwifery.[23] In this instance the reorganisation was prompted by the need to expand and upgrade the institutional framework of the Medical College. The status of midwifery was still marginal in the scheme of scientific medical education owing to its bleak career prospects. Yet the very fact that it was recognised by a separate professorship indicates the beginning of its recognition as a medical discipline.

From the 1850s, the Medical College began to expand its ambit in terms of providing medical training to indigenous male students and chalking out novel ways to accommodate more of them. As scholars have recently pointed out, training indigenous students in western medicine formed one of the keystones in the broader colonial schemes of diffusing western scientific medicine to the lay public. It simultaneously underpinned their civilising mission and the drive to evolve western medicine into a cultural force.[24] To realise these objectives, a Bengali class was started in 1851 and it was further split into two sections in 1864. One of them was a native apothecary section to train students seeking subordinate positions as hospital apprentices in government medical service, in jail hospitals or mostly in charitable dispensaries.[25] The other and more relevant was a vernacular licentiate section to prepare a class of 'minor' indigenous practitioners who were meant to bring the fruits of western scientific medicine to the countryside. The vernacular licentiate class steadily grew in popularity. The spectacular increase in the number of students was proudly cited by the *Indian Medical Gazette* as 'ample proof of the appreciation in which the College Medical education is held by the Natives of Bengal, and how widely the knowledge of European Medicine is spreading throughout the country'.[26]

In 1867, the students of the vernacular class voiced their wish to be instructed in midwifery and the diseases of women and children. Owing to the popularity of this class, the demand of the students struck a chord with J. Ewart, the principal of the Medical College. Ewart considered it imprudent and unwise to inundate the country with minor practitioners bereft of any sound knowledge of midwifery and the diseases of women and children.[27] However, the Medical College Council expressed reluctance in giving the wish of the local students any serious consideration. Dr T. E. Charles, a prominent member of the Council, argued that the practical instructions in midwifery were difficult to carry out due to paucity of actual labour cases. It would eventually have to be accomplished by relying on the prostitutes due to the unavailability of female patients for demonstrative purpose. Emphasising the marginality of midwifery in the medical curriculum of the Bengali class of the Medical College, Dr Charles further stated:

> As regards midwifery I am quite clear that it is a branch of instruction which should be the very last which should be taught to this class of practitioners. When they have a special Teacher of Physiology and a special Teacher of Ophthalmic Medicine, and when all the other elements of a liberal medical education have been provided for, there might be taken into consideration the advisability of instructing them in Midwifery. I would look upon it as absolutely criminal to spend money in teaching them midwifery till all such other wants have been provided for.[28]

Dr Charles's scepticism was part of the contemporary English medical men's perception of midwifery as 'forming a very insignificant portion of the education that a medical man should receive'.[29] In the context of Bengal, however, the predominant reason cited for not promoting midwifery education at the Medical College was the habitual cultural repugnance felt by the Bengali females towards allowing 'manual interference' into their body by male doctors – a fact attested to by the indigenous Sub-Assistant Surgeons themselves.[30] The other more pragmatic reason offered was the hardship encountered in delivering practical instructions in midwifery due to non-availability of labour cases for demonstrative purposes. Hence, in a bid to avoid unnecessary expenditure in instituting separate midwifery training, two of the seven members of the Council suggested the teaching of midwifery by the teachers of medicine and Materia Medica.[31]

The enthusiasm of the students of the licentiate class could not be stemmed by such rebuffs. Agreeing to pay 'Rupees 3 per mensem instead of Rupees 2, provided they were taught midwifery', as many as 155 students out of a class of 188 signed a petition requesting the government to give their wish a serious consideration. Recognising the futility of opposing the demands of the students of this popular vernacular class, the Government of Bengal agreed to the conditional appointment of an additional teacher of midwifery 'as an experimental measure for four months'.[32] Accordingly, a Sub-Assistant Surgeon, Mir Ashraf Ali, who was then a teacher of Medicine at the Agra Medical School, was selected from a group of six candidates, as the teacher of midwifery for the students of the Bengali Licentiate Class of the Medical College. As the official correspondence reveals, the class steadily increased in popularity leading to the post of the teacher of midwifery being eventually made permanent by the Government of India in 1868.[33]

## Training the midwives: a more viable alternative

Following the induction of male students in midwifery class, *Indian Medical Gazette* pessimistically observed that despite a class of Bengali doctors being trained in midwifery at Medical College in the hope of delivering the fruits of 'good midwifery' to the masses, it could assure little benefit to the poor women giving birth in their own homes in distant villages, way beyond the pale of dispensaries/hospitals and the doctors and sub-assistant surgeons attached to them. Thus, it was felt that 'we must advance a step further, and *educate the Native daees themselves*' (emphasis original).[34] However, it was chiefly financial considerations that guided the government in prioritising training of dhais over training of indigenous doctors.

David Arnold argues that replacing the traditional dhais labelled as 'ignorant' and 'barbarous' with trained midwives was a colonial strategy to incorporate women into the 'colonising medical discourse and practice'.[35] Prior to this, the only major colonial intervention in women's health in India had been the passing of the Contagious Diseases Act in 1868 which, following the British Contagious Diseases Act of 1864, provided for the supervision, inspection and treatment of prostitute women in Lock Hospitals. The health of the general Indian population had figured only marginally in colonial health policy till the 1860s, the chief focus being on the army and, at best, the health of the European population. However, the post-1857 transfer of power from the East India Company to the British Crown prompted the restructuring of colonial administration that came to be predicated on a closer consideration of the welfare of the people of India. It was in this political milieu that the colonising and hegemonic potential of western medicine came into fuller view, extending to the sphere of women's health, 'which thereafter assumed a prominent and emblematic position' in the successive debates on the authority of western medicine.[36]

Training of the dhais was, therefore, a major step forward, although the lead had initially been given by women missionaries in several parts of India.[37] In Bengal, the colonial state's effort to educate the dhais, that became visible in the 1860s and 1870s, was more predominantly driven by the logic of sending out 'into native society as large a body of *dhais* as can be procured at a *slight cost to the state*, better trained than those who now act in that capacity' (emphasis mine).[38] Accordingly, a scheme for training the dhais at the Medical College was sanctioned in December 1869 although it was not before the end of December 1870 that a candidate came forward for the training. Later more women 'than could be received' were recorded to have responded favourably to the scheme after advertisements were put up in the English and Bengali newspapers with the help of Brahmo leaders like Keshab Chandra Sen.[39] After a thoughtful consideration, the government approved of a financially viable plan of reducing the number of dhais to be trained from eight to six and placing them under the supervision of a matron. The scheme also provided for their accommodation outside the hospital premises.

The training of female midwives remained one of the key educational planks of the college authorities in the 1870s and 1880s. However, the success of the scheme remained dubious due to the dogged resistance of the dhais to embrace western midwifery practices and the financial constraints of the government. The limited success of the scheme is perhaps a shining example of how the colonial state's attempt to introduce western medicine into the domain of women's health fell flat in the face of its reluctance to finance a sector that was of little direct political or economic interest to the governance of the Empire. That also accounted for the government's overall apathy to Indian women's health throughout the entire colonial period. As Arnold has argued, the colonising potential of western medicine was more fully realised when promoted by the colonised elites themselves.[40]

By the 1880s the educational and practical aspects of midwifery training provided at the Medical College came to be compared with the obstetric hospital in Madras and, to some extent, the Jamshedjee Jeejeebhoy Hospital in Bombay. The proposal for the establishment of a new obstetric hospital within the institutional bounds of the Medical College was floated by Dr Payne, the Surgeon General of Bengal. Madras hospital's remarkable role in sending trained 'native and European' midwives out of the presidency and enabling them to earn their livelihood by private practice was proudly cited in spelling out similar plans for the proposed obstetric hospital in Calcutta.[41] Following the proposal put forward by Dr Payne, the Lieutenant Governor held discussions with Dr Coates and Dr Harvey and, eventually, sanctioned an increased amount to be devoted to the new Obstetric Hospital.[42] The consequence was the founding of the Eden Hospital in Calcutta in July 1882.

The newly established Eden Hospital became the focal point for the training of the dhais. Dr Payne felt that 'no means of replacing the "native" system of midwifery by better practice should be neglected. The teaching of native dhais cannot be sacrificed to that of Europeans and there is no place for it so good as the Eden Hospital'.[43] Yet the number of dhais coming forward for training at the Eden Hospital remained low till the end of the nineteenth century.[44]

Moreover, the paucity of actual labour cases continued to pose a serious constraint on the training in practical obstetrics for male students of the Medical College. Dr Joubert, Professor of midwifery at the Eden Hospital, stated that 'practical instruction in midwifery has always been a great difficulty for the students at the Medical College, and they now only conduct six cases each at the Eden Hospital, and see little or nothing of the treatment of women after labour'.[45] In 1889 Joubert arrived at a solution. Drawing from the example of London hospitals, he proposed the establishment of a Maternity Department. Under such a scheme, women who wished to avail themselves of medical aid could register themselves at the hospital so that they were able to call for assistance on the onset of labour and one of the students attending labour cases would be sent to them. In the case of his failure to handle the case, the 'Resident Obstetric Officer' or the 'Obstetric Physician' would be sent for. Such a scheme would not require women to give birth in the hospitals. It was designed to enable the Medical College students to attend midwifery cases in the homes of the patients. Accordingly, the Lieutenant Governor sanctioned the establishment of a Maternity Department to be attached to the Eden Hospital for one year as an 'experimental measure'.[46]

Such modifications in the structure of midwifery teaching did not immediately indicate expanding professional opportunities for the male doctors choosing to include midwifery in their armoury of knowledge. Training the dhais continued to be the focus of midwifery education instituted at the Medical College. The objective was clearly not to train the dhais in operative midwifery, but to teach them cleanliness and the ability to recognise abnormal labour so that they could promptly seek the help of the doctor. The civil surgeons in Bengal, in charge of training the dhais, were often satisfied if the latter, at the end of three months of training, followed simple rules of hygiene and knew when to seek the assistance of doctor.[47] In view of the fact that the training of dhais was mainly confined to overseeing normal births and, hence, did not serve the needs of female patients needing critical medical attention, a section of medical professionals and some progressive bhadralok increasingly felt the need for a more comprehensive scheme of educating female doctors in India. Yet when compared to the Presidencies of Madras and Bombay, the beginning of female medical education in Bengal was rather shaky and fraught with controversies.

## Female medical education: a step ahead

Following Margaret Balfour and Ruth Young's influential publication, *The work of medical women in India*,[48] scholars have been inclined to focus solely on the contributions of the women medical professionals in drawing Indian women within the ambit of the colonising western medical discourse. Antoinette Burton has argued that providing medical care to Indian women 'imprisoned' in zenana was perceived as a national and an 'imperial obligation' by the British women doctors trained in the London School of Medicine for Women.[49] However, Chandrika Paul has portrayed the entry of Bengali women into the western medical profession as an uneven process, dictated primarily by the individual interests of three groups: British medical women (doctors and missionaries), colonial administrators and the male social reformers (the Brahmos).[50] It is not the intention of this study to question or even belittle the contribution of women doctors in medicalising childbirth. Yet at the same time, it intends to go beyond such exultant historical narratives that pivot on the cliché portrayal of female resistance to male medical aid as the principal factor relegating medicalisation of childbirth to the exclusive control of female doctors. The study aims to identify a wider range of actors in generating the discourse and practice of scientific midwifery. At the same time, it commits to place women doctors in a more nuanced perspective and drive home the point that in attempting to professionalise their sphere of action, the women doctors too ended up echoing the professional ethos of the male-controlled medical structure.

The idea of female medical education had its genesis in the proposal of Dr Balfour, Surgeon General of Madras in 1872. It met with initial opposition from the Madras Medical College authorities, but was eventually supported by the principal of the College. Consequently, four European or Anglo-Indian female students were admitted in 1875. Bombay followed suit. The intervention of an American businessman, George T. Kittredge, led to the Medical Women for India Fund being established in 1880. The Fund laid the groundwork for female medical education and use of medical facilities by women and children in Bombay. In this milieu the Grant Medical College of Bombay eventually opened its door to female candidates in 1883.[51]

In Bengal the proposal traversed a convoluted path of opposition, rejection and acceptance. The delayed response was largely due to bhadralok notions of respectability that led to women's economic independence being seen as a potential threat to the honour of the family. Yet the proposal for admitting women as students in the Medical College was initially made by some progressive Bengalis; for the first time by Babu Neel Kamal Mitra in 1876, then by Rakhal Das Mukherjee in 1879 and finally by parents of two aspiring female candidates, Abala Das and Ellen D'Abreau, in 1882.[52] The proposals were rejected on two grounds by the Calcutta Medical Council.[53] The first reason cited in the *Indian Medical Gazette* was the 'difficulty of introducing a serious innovation into the conservative domain of medical practice'. The second reason was the shortage of funds in promoting the comprehensive scheme of female education.[54]

However, the mediation of a section of progressive Brahmos known as the *Samadarshi Dal* and some well-meaning British administrators such as Alfred Woodley Croft (The Director of Public Instruction), Dr J. M. Coates (Principal of the Medical College) and Rivers

Thompson (Lieutenant Governor of Bengal) led to women being accepted in the Medical College from 1883. Chandrika Paul sees this as an attempt of the British administrative officials to salvage the image of Bengal Presidency and prevent it from falling behind its administrative rivals, Madras and Bombay, in introducing female medical education.[55] Thus, overriding the wave of resistance from the Calcutta Medical Council, Thompson agreed to the admission of female candidates in the Medical College in June 1883. In another resolution dated 6 May 1884, Thompson reemphasised the policy of female education by offering scholarships to those female candidates who, after successfully qualifying for the First Arts Examination at the University, would be 'elected' as students at the Medical College. His endeavour was greatly bolstered by the munificence of Maharani Swarnamayi who donated a considerable sum of money to the Government of Bengal to be utilised in whichever way possible. The consequence was the construction of a hostel for the accommodation of Indian female medical students.[56] The earliest beneficiary was Kadambini Basu who was awarded the GBMC (Graduate of Bengal Medical College) in 1886.

The college authorities proposed an arrangement wherein the women students should be screened off from the male candidates. The study of anatomical details of naked human form challenged the gender hierarchy and patriarchal order that had strong resonances in the conservative British society in the nineteenth century. However, women's consent to sit in 'mixed classes' with men heralded the beginning of women's entrance into the professional sphere of obstetrics and gynaecology, a fact that became evident with the foundation of the Dufferin Fund.

The Countess of Dufferin Fund was the short-hand for the 'National Association for Supplying Female Medical Aid to the Women of India' named after the Vicereine Lady Dufferin. The Fund was a landmark in the institutionalisation of midwifery in India. As a semi-official effort, its origin was linked to the women's movement in Britain. It was established to provide 'medical relief to women by women, medical tuition of women and the doing of all things conducive to these objects'. The Fund prompted the establishment and expansion of an intricate network of female hospitals, dispensaries and clinics on city and district levels with branches in all major cities of India. The branches were supervised and managed by a Central Committee composed of powerful Englishmen and wealthy Indian aristocrats (male and female) and presided over by the Vicereine.[57]

The importance of the Fund lay in the impetus it gave to the study of midwifery in colonial India. Within two years of the establishment of the Fund, the Government of Bengal ratified the recruitment of female students to the Bengali class of the Campbell Medical School for medical instruction on exactly similar lines designed for 'Civil Hospital Assistants'. The requirements for admission were relaxed and pushed to a lower level for the female students. The prospective female hospital assistants were trained with a view to enabling them to practise in the villages and districts of Bengal. In 1892, the standard of female professional education was raised by the Government of Bengal when it resolved to introduce University Entrance Examination as the criterion for admission and increased the period of study from three to four years for certificate classes.[58]

By 1895, 24 women students were enrolled in the classes of the CMC and a further 34 of them were attending the hospital assistant class of the Campbell Medical School.[59] While the alleged discriminatory and racist nature of employment policies practised under the Fund was grudged in the Bengali press,[60] the Fund-operated dispensaries and hospitals in districts provided increased employment opportunities for licentiate female doctors as hospital assistants and, as Geraldine Forbes has argued, aided the spread of western medical treatment into the districts of Bengal.[61] Thus, paradoxically enough, female licentiate doctors being denied lucrative jobs in urban hospitals played a major role in popularising western medicine in the districts.

The Dufferin Fund also took care to extend 'hospital habits' amongst the purdahnashin women. In order to attract more patients, concerns were voiced in the Annual Reports of the Bengal branch of the Fund regarding the increasing necessity to secure the privacy of the wards. Attention had to be paid to the 'details of cook-houses, store-rooms, arrangements for the accommodation of the friends of patients and for members of the hospital staff and establishment. . . . Much may yet be accomplished to obtain greater privacy in existing institutions'.[62] The Eurasian, Christian, Jew and Armenian female population was excluded from the scope of medical treatment provided at the purdah hospitals and male civil surgeons were later barred from inspecting the purdah wards.[63] The 'secular' nature of the medical work discharged by the Fund was repeatedly asserted. Every attempt towards dissociating itself from the missionaries and the overtly religious nature of their work was prioritised and implemented.[64] Yet the attendance of Hindu purdahnashin women remained low.[65]

However, at the turn of the century, the trend of women seeking western medical care in the Dufferin Fund–operated hospitals escalated although the patients were not necessarily Hindu purdahnashins.[66] In the process, the line of demarcation between what constituted a

Dufferin Fund–operated hospital and what in reality was a female ward of a general hospital often became blurred. For instance, it was revealed in the seventeenth annual report of the Dufferin Fund in 1904 that increasing number of women and children in many parts of Lower Bengal were being treated by the civil surgeons in the general hospitals and dispensaries maintained by local funds rather than by the Dufferin Fund. Being assisted by female hospital assistants and dhais, the bulk of the treatment was administered by the civil surgeon. In this context, the *Indian Medical Gazette* pointed out,

> in a score of instances, and there may be others, the work done in general hospitals in the districts is simply incorporated with that done in special Dufferin Hospitals and classed as the latter. Thus, it would seem to appear that in Lower Bengal a large number of the women and children medically treated by Government officials are regarded as relief afforded by the Dufferin Fund.[67]

While this resulted in women doctors being controlled by male civil surgeons leading to recurring resentments amongst the former, the appeal of the 'female' hospitals promising to secure the modesty of the Bengali women often drew women, some of whom were also non-purdahnashin, to such hospitals. Also the presence of Bengali female hospital assistants like Haimabati Sen in charge of the Hooghly Dufferin Hospital and Hemangini Devi in charge of the Dufferin Victoria Hospital in Bankura contributed significantly towards attracting local female patients.[68]

However, the female doctors faced persistent challenges of having to compete with the male civil surgeons in the sphere of actual practice in the dispensaries and hospitals. Consequently, they sought to appropriate all those arenas of medical practice which were hitherto controlled and monopolised by male physicians. The rationale driving their demand for autonomy and recognition was, 'A medical woman who intends to work among Indian women must be *better qualified* than a man engaged in medical work out here, *not less qualified*' (emphasis original).[69] In the case of Bengal, it resulted in a tussle between the civil surgeons and the 'lady doctors'. One of the crucial areas of contest was surgery. The long-standing taboo against women performing surgery had been one of the major considerations of the male-dominated medical establishment in Bengal in allowing the civil surgeons to perform major operations. The civil surgeons were wary of the prospects of not having 'excellent surgery' in female hospitals and the chances of losing control over the appointments of women hospital assistants.[70]

As Margaret Balfour stated in her account, despite women doctors sometimes 'not being personally keen on surgery', surgery was still perceived by them as a crucial way to refine medical training and enhance the status of the female hospitals.[71]

The later reports of the Dufferin Fund testify to an increasing number of women doctors performing surgical operations. To cite an example, the report of the Bengal branch of the Dufferin Fund showed Haimabati Sen, a Hospital Assistant at the Hooghly Dufferin Hospital, performing four craniotomies and seven forceps deliveries in the year 1895, the number steadily increasing in the following years with Sen being in 'sole' charge of a wide variety of 'operations' in the hospital and the outpatient clinic.[72] Further the Inspector General of Civil Hospitals, Bengal confirmed in August 1910 that the number of abdominal operations in Dufferin Hospital in Calcutta had gone up from ten in 1907 to eighty in 1908 and fifty-seven in 1909, also describing the operation room as small but 'well-equipped'.[73] It might be argued here that the presumed fear of Indians for surgery was greatly allayed by the female doctors who in wielding surgical instruments broke all taboos and popularised western medical practice.

In a bid to foster their professional interests, the female medical practitioners formed the Association of Medical Women in India in Bombay in 1907 with divisions established in each of the states in India. Yet, it was mostly the British female doctors and not their Indian counterparts who pursued an aggressive propaganda for acquiring greater professional recognition than men in the sphere of obstetrics and gynaecology.[74] The first president of the Association, Dr Annette Benson (from the Cama Hospital Bombay), argued that the medical women in India were

> nondescript scattered members of isolated units, at the mercy of chance employment and still more chance conditions of service, and almost all in subordinate positions . . . we aim so to improve the conditions under which the medical women work as to make their work efficient and their reward fair.[75]

In 1911 – precisely at a juncture when medical women's demands for a Women's Medical Service (WMS) in India were about to be fulfilled – Kathleen O' Vaughan argued that Indian women preferred to be attended by female doctors than by male ones only if the former were equally competent. 'Indian' female doctors would still be more preferable provided they were 'well qualified' and 'well educated'.[76]

Being affiliated to the International Association of Medical Women, the Association for Medical Women in India was conceived as a fulcrum for the transnational exchange of knowledge, experiences and research of medical women. Soon, the Association joined hands with the Central Committee of the Dufferin Fund in making two representations to the Government of India in 1910 and 1912 petitioning the formation of a covenanted women's medical service along the lines of the IMS.[77] The second representation succeeded and in 1913 the Government of India sanctioned the grant of an increased subsidy of one and a half lakh rupees to the Central Committee of the Dufferin Fund that led to the foundation of the WMS on 1 January 1914.[78] The WMS underscored an all India basis for the organisation of women's medical work in providing improved hospital services and better quality medical aid to women.

In competing with their male counterparts and clamouring for greater professional status, the women doctors ended up appropriating male professional ethos.[79] In recent times, scholars like Nancy M. Theriot have nudged us to premise our historical enquiries on the more balanced concept of gender and science being 'mutually constitutive'.[80] Further Regina Markell Morantz-Sanchez's historical study of women physicians in the American medical profession in the twentieth century has revealed 'therapeutic similarities' in the treatment rendered by male and women physicians. To quote Morantz-Sanchez,

> women physicians were not only women, but physicians as well. As physicians, they operated under the dictates of their profession: they viewed themselves as full-fledged health professionals, they read the same journals as the men, and they subscribed to theories that they believed represented the collected wisdom of their group.[81]

In India, in the interwar years (as Chapter 3 will demonstrate) need to lower maternal and infant mortality provided a powerful impetus to constitute obstetrics and gynaecology into a more cohesive profession that could not always be rigidly demarcated along gender lines.

The thrust was not on 'more doctors' but 'better doctors' with 'wider medical outlook' and greater 'scientific spirit'; women physicians had to 'keep abreast of modern methods and continually improve their standard of practice'.[82] Professional competence was cited as one of the preconditions for treating more female patients and, more significantly, for marginalising male medical professionals in the domain of obstetrics. This was further backed by the demands of the Indian women's organisations in the 1930s that maternity homes and maternal and child welfare clinics be placed under the exclusive charge of women doctors, health visitors and trained midwives.[83]

Recognising the need for greater coordination between male and female medical professionals in obstetrics, the renowned obstetrician from Madras L. S. Mudaliar suggested three ways to do it at the Obstetric section of the tenth All India Medical Conference held in 1934: (a) introducing postgraduate training in the subject, (b) promoting original 'clinical research' in diseases associated with pregnancy or 'tropical' diseases complicating pregnancy and (c) founding associations that would infuse great interest amongst the obstetricians and gynaecologists practising the 'twin arts' and promote the profession.[84]

Mudaliar's endeavours led to the establishment of the Madras Obstetric and Gynaecological Society in 1934. Bengal followed suit and founded a similar association in 1936. The founding of such provincial professional associations was followed by holding of annual Congresses as a means to 'unite the whole obstetric profession in India in a body to achieve the status and exert influence as it is in other countries of the world'.[85] While the first Obstetric and Gynaecological Congress was organised in the city of Madras in 1936 and the second in Bombay in 1937, the third was held in Bengal in 1941. Not only was the membership of the Society and participation in the Congress opened to both male and female physicians, it was also iterated in the presidential address that in order to ensure efficiency and wide accessibility of midwifery services,

> the man-midwife – as he was called in derision – has to work in company of a lady-midwife. If both are efficient, if they do their work in harmony, readily and willingly co-operating with each other . . . they would prove to be benevolent angels to villagers.[86]

Female obstetricians and physicians contributed papers at the Congress and enriched the discussion on pathological aspects of pregnancy and on efficient ways of conducting maternity benefit schemes. Their engagement with scientific research on maternal diseases and other aspects of women's gynaecological health conducted under the auspices of the Indian Research Fund Association or the AIIHPH intensified in the interwar years and thereafter.

## 'Male' doctors in the 'Female' domain of midwifery[87]

In a recent work, Monica H. Green has asserted the role of men in childbirth in the West, arguing 'that they were "hiding in plain sight" more often than we suspect'.[88] Drawing upon Green's argument and expanding it further, this section argues that the role of male physicians in effecting transformations in the knowledge and practice of midwifery was of a significant nature and hence deserves closer analysis.

The inadequacy of historical research on the agency of male physicians in medicalisation of childbirth in India throws open an unexplored field of enquiry. At the same time, the lack of primary documents poses the formidable challenge of collating and reconstructing a narrative from an array of diverse and scattered sources. Acknowledging this constraint, the book chose to liberally draw upon a huge gamut of medical journals: official ones like the *Indian Medical Gazette* and the non-official and privately run ones, such as the *Calcutta Medical Journal, the Indian Medical Record* and the *Journal of the Indian Medical Association*.[89] Equally vital has been the copious use of vernacular medical journals like *Bishak Darpan, Cikitsa Prakasa, Cikitsa Sammilani* in analysing the contours of an evolving medical discourse on midwifery that found expression in print from the late nineteenth century onwards.

In a recent extensive study on medicalisation of childbirth in colonial Bengal, Supriya Guha has argued that 'the obstetric revolution that had taken place in England in the eighteenth and nineteenth centuries was brought to India by mainly medical women'.[90] The term 'obstetric revolution' coined by Irvine Loudon loosely referred to the emergence of 'man-midwife' or male accoucheurs in England between 1730 and 1770, whose 'scientific proficiency' and possession of the 'forceps' not only threatened the traditional roles of midwives as birth attendants but also led to a 'reformulation of the ideological basis of midwifery'.[91] Drawing upon this definition of what constituted 'obstetric revolution' there is much truth in Guha's argument about the palpable absence of a category of 'man-midwife' in the early history of medicalisation of childbirth in Bengal. Yet a closer analysis unfolds how the process of incorporation of midwifery into the medical curriculum of the CMC was inextricably associated with its re-inscription in medical terms. The process of re-inscription was effected to a considerable extent through the intervention of male medical practitioners.

Two distinct patterns of male physicians' engagement with the domain of obstetrics constitute the theme of this analysis: first, the position of male doctors as general practitioners within an emerging *daktari* culture in mid nineteenth-century Bengal. This chapter analyses how general practitioners practising midwifery in the districts sought to appropriate western medical discourse on childbirth both in terms of learning midwifery and attending actual cases of childbirth. Second, the chapter locates the male specialists or obstetricians within a more expanded domain of professionalised obstetrics that drew heavily on the national and the global. The chapter seeks to demonstrate how the exposure of the obstetricians to the medical education in the West endowed them with a more nuanced understanding of the discipline of obstetrics.

The indigenous male physician's involvement in childbirth can be located in a new pattern of medical culture or *daktari* that evolved in mid-nineteenth-century Bengal. In a recent extensive historical work on the subject, Projit Behari Mukharji has defined *daktari* as a 'self-descriptive category' that increasingly gained currency in the 1860s and came to embody a distinctive set of practices, separate from the existing indigenous systems of medicine. *Daktari* underscored a dual process of 'provincialisation' and 'vernacularisation' of western medicine that was enabled by three trends: the nationalisation of Ayurveda as the quintessential Hindu medical system by the western writers in the 1830s and 1840s that led to the provincialisation of allopathy as the product of the West, the gradual marginalisation of Bengali Sub-Assistant Surgeon by the colonial government after the 1860s and, lastly, the opening of the Bengali licentiate class at the Medical College that generated demand for Bengali books and periodicals.[92] *Daktari* underscored the translation of European medical texts into Bengali and the creation of Bengali medical vocabulary through adoption of western medical terms. One of the central features of Daktari practice in Bengal, according to Mukharji, was the constant need to 'nationalise' and 'de-alienate' itself from the masses by incorporating local customs and cultural beliefs into its medical repertoire.[93] Mukharji has further explained how the identity and social meanings of *daktari* were constantly contested and negotiated in the Bengali printing world through periodicals, advertisements and drama.

It was through the medium of vernacular medical periodicals, the *daktars* developed and disseminated a western scientific discourse on midwifery in Bengali language.[94] However, the *daktars* engaging in midwifery were clearly more predisposed towards embracing western medical approach to childbirth than incorporating local medical traditions and seeking a harmonious mingling of the two. As has been discussed in Chapter 1, the diffusion of a prescriptive scientific body of knowledge on midwifery was carried initially through the pages of women's journals like *Bamabodhini Patrika* from the 1860s. It reflected a certain degree of social commitment towards expurgating ignorance and irrationality from the female domain of midwifery and also formed a powerful way of spreading the gospel of modern medicine to the inner quarters of home. This section will analyse how a 'medical' view of childbirth was discursively constructed in the pages of vernacular medical journals and later dispersed through individual compositions on pregnancy and the diseases of women.

Dr Annada Charan Khastagir's 'A Treatise on the Science and Practice of Midwifery with Diseases of Children and Women' was one of the earliest and fruitful attempts to redefine midwifery as a medical discipline.[95] Khastagir was the Sub-Assistant Surgeon under the IMS. The centrality of his text lay in its dual commitment to serve the needs of the 'native doctors of the Bengali class and the students of the medical schools' and to engage in meaningful dialogue with the indigenous systems of medicines by incorporating local (*desiya*) treatment within the ambit of discussion.[96] Being originally written in 1868, it was one of the earliest texts that brought intricate diagrammatic and theoretical details of obstetric surgical instruments such as forceps, vectis and fillets into the scope of discussion. It also vividly illustrated and evaluated the pros and cons of important obstetric operations such as craniotomy, symphisiotomy, episiotomy, version and caesarean section. Similar treatises belonging to this genre included Khirodaprasad Chattopadhyay's *Dhatribidya* ('Art of Midwifery') and Nagendranath Sengupta's *Sochitro Daktari Siksha* ('An Illustrated Treatise on Allopathic Medicine').[97] Such monographs continued to be published sporadically throughout the nineteenth century and signalled the existence of a well-entrenched *daktari* practice in Bengal.

However, it was with the publication of vernacular medical journals from the 1880s and the 1890s that sustained intellectual discourse/dialogue on the medical aspects of midwifery along with other specialised branches of medical science became a possibility for the Bengali *daktars* trained in western medicine. In 1888, Dr Jadunath Gangopadhyay pressed the need for medical associations of Bengali medical men (in Calcutta and mufassils) and medical journals written in Bengali language as the most effective ways to eradicate ignorance and ensure improved circulation of medical knowledge amongst the Bengali physicians.[98] Arguing along similar lines, the inaugural issue of *Cikitsa Prakasa* (Health Highlights) in 1909 stated that:

> In order to excel in medical care and treatment, it is essential to acquire knowledge in various directions and subjects related to

medical science . . . the saddest thing is that the doctors in our country being ignorant of the English language are deprived of the opportunity to acquire knowledge on various subjects. Lack of contemporary medical periodicals in Bengali language is the main reason for this constraint.[99]

The journal laid out four objectives: (1) to publish important extracts from contemporary English medical journals; (2) to publish important research findings of experienced medical men; (3) to provide detailed description of theories of various diseases; and (4) detailed analysis of specific ailments.[100] Much of what was published in the pages of the vernacular medical journals was directly linked to the creation and consolidation of a professional identity for the licentiate doctors in Bengal. Quite evidently therefore, the readership of these journals was usually confined to the medical community: the *daktars* in particular. The publication of such journals enabled unimpeded dissemination of western medical knowledge in Bengali language amongst the teachers and students of vernacular licentiate class.

Prior to the publication of *Cikitsa Prakasa* quite a few medical periodicals such as *Cikitsa Sammilani, Svasthya, Anubikshan, Cikitsa Darpan* and *Bishak Darpan* had already been in circulation since the last two decades of the nineteenth century. Particularly significant was *Bishak Darpan* that derived financial support from the government and remained in circulation for a fairly long period of time. *Bishak Darpan* provided a forum for exchanging and acquiring specialised knowledge in various fields of medical science within the ambit of western system of medicine. It included important essays on midwifery as well.

By the 1890s in England, midwifery had emerged from the fringes of medical profession into one of the core aspects of medical training. In the 1880s, medical men practising in London and other suburban hospitals could boast of having

> gained our knowledge of distortions of the pelvis; we have a clearer appreciation of the condition of uterus in obstructed labour . . . we have gained in the more frequent and earlier use of forceps, in our safer management of the third stage of labour . . . in our methods of dealing with haemorrhage . . . in our acquaintance with puerperal eclampsia, embolism, and thrombosis.[101]

The evolution of gynaecology as the necessary adjunct to obstetrics led to the further expansion of the ambit of the discipline, indicating the growing importance of surgery in the medical management of birth. This caused a section of the British obstetricians to express concerns about the abuse of the knowledge of surgery and the consequent contamination of the 'natural' process of childbirth[102] reminiscent of similar anti-interventionist debates in the eighteenth century.[103] The weight of the debate in the nineteenth century had tilted more heavily in favour of judicious medical supervision and intervention in childbirth. Such debates found resonance in the medical journals in Bengal in the late nineteenth and early twentieth centuries.

The essays which appeared in *Bishak Darpan* were essentially translated versions of important writings by British doctors or, in certain instances, individual compositions of LMS or VLMS degree holders[104] who derived much of what they wrote from the writings of British medical professionals. The predominant focus of the writings was on the pathological aspects of labour and post-pregnancy maladies such as placenta praevia, post-partum haemorrhage, puerperal fever etc. The central point of emphasis was, however, the need for 'discreet' use of modern methods of treatment available to the practitioners of midwifery, cautions being made against 'meddlesome midwifery'.[105] 'Puerperal Fever' known in Bengal as '*Sutikajor*' is a case in point. At a time when puerperal fever constituted the most menacing threat to the women giving birth in England and was considered the 'plague which haunts the whole domain of midwifery',[106] conflicting ideas regarding the origin of the disease that were intensely debated in England found resonance in the writings of Bengali medical men. The new notion was that the disease was a form of 'obstetric poisoning' either caused by pus formation within the body or introduced from outside by the unskilled surgeon's 'careless surgical dressing' or the midwife's unclean hands. Such ideas trickled down to the pages of Bengali medical journals that also acknowledged hospitals as the point of origin of puerperal fever.[107] An essay entitled 'Duties towards a Parturient Woman' written by a licentiate doctor, Rameshchandra Roy, spelt out certain measures to combat puerperal fever such as 'surgical cleanliness', the need to maintain antiseptic conditions throughout the three stages of labour and also the need to avoid 'douching'. Roy also critiqued the 'unhygienic' conditions of birth in Bengali homes, considering it as one of the chief causes for puerperal fever.[108] Explicit connections between 'unhygienic' sutikaghar and puerperal fever were also made in the women's magazines at the turn of the century.[109]

*Cikitsa Prakasa* published individual accounts of indigenous male physicians serving in the districts of Bengal under the title of *Cikitsitorogirbiboron* ('Description of a Treated Patient'). It is interesting to note how the indigenous doctors claimed the superiority and 'proven effectiveness' of the allopathic line of treatment over the indigenous methods. One of them posted in Rangilabad Hooghly (a district in Bengal) described his intervention as being extremely timely in saving the life of a woman stuck with a dead foetus for three days. He denounced the damage caused by the unskilled midwife and the irrational folk treatment of 'warding off evil spirit', and claimed his remedies (the allopathic medicines he administered) to be crucial in bringing her back to life.[110]

At the turn of the century, individual compositions on scientific midwifery by licentiate male doctors that had already been in vogue in the 1860s and 1870s gained renewed prominence. Despite having technological components and clear-cut scientific perspectives, such tracts were written in lucid Bengali in order to attract popular readership, being directed both at the midwives and the middle-class readers. For instance, Abhaya Kumar Sarkar's *Prasuti Paricharya o Sisu Palan* ('Treatment of the Pregnant Woman and Infant Rearing') was published with the objective of instructing the dhais in the training centres located in the districts of Bengal and also to enlighten the middle-class women, the newly married women and the elderly housewives on scientific details of labour and childbearing. According to the Health Officer of the Calcutta Corporation, the book was of great value to the middle-class women who wished to know more about midwifery 'for the sake of their own health'.[111] It was lucid enough for the use of half-educated village women as well.[112] The book was showered with praises by the medical fraternity and the nationalist press. *Amrita Bazar Patrika* evaluated its importance 'in the light of the valuable information it furnishes its readers about fundamental principles of obstetrics and gynaecology, so far as these principles can be explained in Bengali language'.[113]

Similarly, Devendranatha Roy's *Garhasthya Svasthyaraksha o sochitro dhatrisiksha* ('Domestic Hygiene and Illustrated Guide to Midwifery') published in 1904 was a detailed attempt to propagate revised scientific rules related to childbirth and prescribed interventionist approach in conducting complicated labour. Roy was a licentiate doctor and having served as a teacher of medical jurisprudence and hygiene at the Campbell Medical School and also having already written a book on the subject, '*Sochitro Dhatrisiksha*' was his second important composition. Written in the form of a dialogue between the master and the pupil *Sochitro Dhatrisiksha* chose to convey the most baffling aspects of the subject in a lucid and intelligible manner.[114] Such genre of easily readable medical tracts and monographs on reproductive health and childbirth continued to proliferate reaching its peak in the 1930s.[115]

The Bengali tracts on midwifery often merged with another distinct genre of writings on gynaecological ailments published under the title of '*Stri Cikitsa*'(treatment of females) that were intended for 'home' use.[116] In certain instances, other existing medical discourses such as homeopathy and Ayurveda on midwifery and diseases of women found their way into this genre of medical writings. For instance, in the homeopathic reproductive manual entitled '*Stri Cikitsa*'(treatment of women) the author Radha Raman Sarkar's advocacy of homeopathy over allopathic system of medicine was founded on a comparison of 'simple', 'non-surgical' homeopathic remedies with the presumed complexities of the allopathic mode of treatment based on frequent recourse to forceps application and craniotomy.[117] Similarly, Ayurveda tracts on midwifery and gynaecology made claims about healing women's diseases in harmony with indigenous traditions.[118] Such competing medical discourses that jostled with each other indicated the struggle of the male physicians to penetrate the zenana through printed words.

However, the sphere of activities of the *daktar* was circumscribed by lack of original research, being mostly based on inherited knowledge from the West. Also the practice being confined to district dispensaries, the scope for experimenting with the more advanced form of operative obstetrics such as caesarean section and other newly evolved techniques from the West was limited. Herein the role of specialists or obstetricians as opposed to the more local and less qualified general practitioner or *daktars* demands closer historical focus.

## The rise of the obstetricians

The specialisation of the male 'obstetricians' in the field of obstetrics and their appointment as professors of midwifery underscored the beginning of an enduring engagement with improving midwifery education and the broadening of the ambit of clinical–scientific research in the 'tropical' specificities of midwifery. The association of these obstetricians or 'specialists' with Calcutta-based major teaching hospitals and medical schools put them in possession of key organisational resources. The career of Dr Kedarnath Das who was referred to by the *Amrita Bazar Patrika* as a great obstetrician, a 'gifted physician and a profound scholar in medical science' in India serves as a key example in tracing the agency of male obstetricians in regulating the domain of birth in Bengal.[119]

On Kedarnath Das's death in 1936, his colleague V. B. Green-Armytage summed up his accomplishments in the following words:

> Kedarnath Das was India's greatest obstetric guru, for he was the first Indian to call attention to the need of Western methods for stemming its dreadful maternal and infantile mortality; and this he did on the platform and in books and journals for forty years.[120]

Das graduated from the CMC in 1892 and also acquired an MD degree from Madras in 1895. Beginning with the position of Medical and Surgical Registrar at the Medical College, he moved on to become a teacher at Campbell Medical School in Sealdah which placed him on the list of Civil Assistant Surgeons. Das's position put him in charge of major obstetrics operations.[121] He ended up becoming the professor of obstetrics and gynaecology and the principal of the Carmichael College in 1922. He held key administrative positions as the dean of the Faculty of Medicine at the Calcutta University, as a member of the Bengal Council of Medical Registration and even as part of the governing body of the State Medical Faculty of Bengal. He also enjoyed the privileged membership of the American Association of Obstetricians, Gynaecologists and Abdominal Surgeons and the Foundation Fellowship of the British College of Obstetricians and Gynaecologists. He was granted a knighthood in 1933.[122]

Kedarnath Das's claim to fame, as evident in the designations he held and the membership of the associations he enjoyed, lay chiefly in the way he redefined midwifery in the language of surgery. Das's use of forceps as one of the linchpins of modern midwifery led him to compose what has been acknowledged as his greatest work entitled *Obstetric Forceps: Its History and Evolution* published in 1928. Being a product of twelve years of fruitful research, *Obstetric Forceps* was grounded in his conviction that forceps was a 'noble and beneficent instrument, rescuing more lives and cutting short more pains than all other instruments in the professional armamentarium'.[123] Prior to this, Das found out by pelvimetry (measurement of the pelvis) that the pelvis of the Bengali woman was much smaller than those of the British woman. The small size of the pelvis along with the fact that Bengali women conceived at a relatively young age owing to the deep-rooted social custom of child marriage made the use of forceps manufactured according to British standards both inappropriate and fatal upon the women of Bengal. This prompted Das to modify the ordinary Simpson type of forceps so as to make it 'fit' for use in Bengali women. What he eventually came up with was the remodelled 'Bengal Forceps' that was in great use since 1913 by himself and other Bengali practitioners. It was claimed to be 'more useful and less harmful in Bengali women than the other usual types obtainable at the surgical instrument makers' shop'.[124] In the process, the 'noble' and 'beneficent' aspects of the instrument were successfully retained.

Prior to Das's work, detailed description of forceps is also to be found, as mentioned before, in Annada Charan Khastagir's 'A Treatise on the Science and Practice of Midwifery with Diseases of Children and Women' and in other such stray monographs published in the 1860s and 1870s. None of them indicated however the incidence of forceps delivery in Bengal or the extent of its popularity amongst the middle class. The Annual reports of the Bengal branch of the Dufferin Fund from the 1890s onwards point towards forceps delivery by the civil surgeons and the women hospital assistants in the district hospitals of Bengal. By the 1920s, forceps was popularly perceived as an instrument designed to relieve women from the pangs of prolonged labour. As one doctor stated, one of the reasons behind the high incidence of forceps in Calcutta hospitals was the implorings of the patient and her 'oversympathetic relations' to the surgeon or the midwife in attendance that labour be terminated by the use of forceps.[125]

Following Das, debates on the place of forceps in obstetrics continued to figure in indigenous medical circles.[126] Individual compositions by Bengali doctors in the 1930s and 1940s however sought to relegate the use of forceps to the 'specialised' professional domain deeming it as a 'safe instrument, in the hands of a skilful accoucheur . . . a dangerous weapon in the hands of a person who is not accustomed to its proper use'.[127]

Das's nationalist sensibilities prodded him to seek out the 'Hindu' roots of surgery. In repudiating the western origin of surgery, Das asserted that

> one may reasonably observe that Indian medicine was in possession of an imposing treasure of empirical knowledge and technical achievement . . . surgery constituted the summit of attainment of Indian medicine and Hindu practitioners were accustomed to perform difficult operations with boldness and skill.[128]

Also as a professor of midwifery, he sought to improve the standards of education in midwifery through writing two prominent and popular instructive manuals entitled *A Handbook of Obstetrics* (1914) and *A Textbook of Midwifery* (1920) for the use of medically trained doctors.[129]

Das's contribution to obstetrics, therefore, lay in his effort to adapt western medical ideas to local Bengali conditions. There were still other Bengali male obstetricians who sought to modernise and technologise the sphere of Indian midwifery through emulation of western techniques, but carefully linked such techniques to certain aspects of past 'Hindu' medical practices in order to ensure greater acceptability. To cite an example, J. M. Das, the resident surgeon in the Eden Hospital and also the officiating teacher of midwifery at the Campbell Medical School, undertook an experiment in 1917 on patients admitted to the Eden Hospital. He experimented with the use of 'scopolamine and morphine narcosis' – the scientific term for 'twilight sleep' – on fifty patients (including Europeans and Bengalis) with the 'most gratifying results'.[130] These drugs which were intended to be deployed as anaesthetics for alleviating pain in childbirth were opposed in the press in Bengal. The controversy caused great inconvenience to the surgeons and medical staff in the Eden Hospital.[131] However, Das argued in favour of 'twilight sleep' by stating:

> Attempts to relieve the pains of labour date back to antiquity. In the dim past we find that the Hindoos used to exorcise the pangs of motherhood by means of the vapour of charcoal which had the effect of stupefying the senses . . . if surgeons will not permit their patients to suffer during an operation why should not an obstetrician mitigate the sufferings of childbirth taking the necessary precautions that no ill effects come to the mother or to the child?[132]

The advocacy of the use of scopolamine and morphine in childbirth could also possibly have emanated from the professional concerns to intensify control over the birthing process by drawing women within the hospital structure that enabled the use of such anaesthetics and offering more to women in labour than the dhai or midwife could.

In the twentieth century, the discovery and deployment of the techniques of blood transfusion (1906) and chemotherapy aided the expansion of the technological and operative domain of obstetrics in England and America. Echoes of such developments came to redefine the priorities of the burgeoning medical profession in Bengal. The spotlight was now on experimenting with advanced techniques of surgery in obstetrics under the pretext of curbing maternal and foetal mortality. In fact, medical profession's expansion in India was premised upon experimenting with upgraded medical and technological accomplishments in other countries and applying them to indigenous situations. In this context, the minister in charge of Local Self Government

(Medical Department) Bijoy Krishna Singh Roy argued that one of the goals of training officers of the Bengal Medical Service abroad was

> to enable them to acquire first-hand knowledge of the latest developments in the art and science of medicine, including medical education, in Western countries and to acquaint themselves with the latest methods of dealing with hospital work and medical relief in general and the problems appertaining thereto as practised in Western countries.[133]

Of all the evolved techniques of obstetric surgery, caesarean section came in for a lot of critical analysis in the pages of the Indian medical journals from the second decade of the twentieth century. In the 1920s, Bengali doctors felt that C-section was 'an operation which is having an ever widening application in the complications of pregnancy, and should and undoubtedly before long will replace many of the complicated and risky manipulations at present practised'.[134] Being consigned to the domain of the specialists, it was considered an intricate operation calling for 'unquestionable operative abilities' and 'good obstetric judgment' which the general practitioner lacked.[135] Towards the end of the 1920s, the more advanced techniques of C-section evolved in America and elsewhere and made inroads into the medical vocabulary of obstetric practice in Bengal. Thus, V. B. Green-Armytage, the professor of midwifery at the Eden Hospital, urged the importance of lower segment caesarean section developed by Professor De Lee in Chicago. He advised the female hospitals entirely staffed by women doctors to learn the technique. He testified to 75 cases of lower-uterine segment caesarean section being personally performed by him from 1927 to 1931 at the Eden Hospital, apart from there being 163 instances of the same operation conducted in the same institution with very little maternal and foetal mortality.[136] M. V. Webb, a female superintendent in charge of the Victoria Zenana Hospital in Hyderabad, testified to the growing popularity of surgical intervention in obstetric practice throughout the country since the first decade of the twentieth century. The factors enabling greater surgical intervention, according to Webb, were the 'greater confidence' of people in surgery, the 'increased ease of transport' and, lastly, the 'increased confidence of the surgeons' in endorsing surgical interventions as the 'safest' mode of delivery.[137]

By the 1930s, male obstetricians had made significant inroads into the professionalised domain of midwifery both in terms of the research attempted and also in applying improved techniques learnt from the West to the Bengali conditions. In promoting advanced operative techniques like C-section and in pleading for non-operative experimental measures like 'twilight sleep', the Bengali doctors were voicing the need to upgrade obstetrics and fortify its scientific foundations in keeping with international standards. In the 1930s, new teaching hospitals such as the Carmichael Medical College were established apart from several medical schools in Calcutta and in the districts of Jalpaiguri, Burdwan, Bankura, Dacca, Mymensingh and Chittagong, all imparting training in midwifery. Nevertheless, as the last section will show, the practical training in midwifery for the male students continued to pose a serious challenge for the existing pedagogic framework of the Calcutta University. The difficulty of practical training fuelled by the paucity of labour cases led to the withdrawal of recognition of Indian medical degrees by the General Medical Council of the United Kingdom in 1924. The issue, as the last section will demonstrate, had a profound impact on the consolidation of nationalist sentiments amongst the male doctors.

## Midwifery and nationalism

The medical degrees of the Calcutta University ceased to be recognised on 30 November 1924 under a resolution of the General Council of Medical Education and Registration (GMC) of the United Kingdom. The unsatisfactory nature of training in midwifery imparted at the Indian Universities was cited as one of the major reasons behind the decision. Consequently, persons obtaining MB (Bachelor of Medicine) degrees after 30 November 1924 would not only cease to be entitled to registration for the 'Colonial List of Medical Registers' but also be debarred from obtaining higher qualifications in the United Kingdom. Already in 1920, the authorities of the Calcutta University were informed that unless adequate measures were adopted in bringing the training up to 'the requisite standard by a fixed date, Calcutta University medical qualifications would cease to be registrable in the United Kingdom'.[138] Lieutenant Colonel Needham was appointed by the Medical Council as the Official Inspector. He was, however, refused permission by the Vice Chancellor of the Calcutta University and the Syndicate to inspect the MB examinations. Based on Needham's reports, the GMC terminated the recognition of the medical degrees of the Calcutta University in 1924, while it continued to recognise degrees of other Indian universities until 1930.

On a broader level, the central point of the Medical Council's threat to the Indian Universities lay chiefly in the way it afforded opportunities for the members of the IMS to retain control over the medical colleges. As Roger Jeffery has aptly argued, it also enabled the IMS to 'reduce the number of students admitted, toughen up the conditions for passing examinations, retain more of the lucrative medical college jobs than they might otherwise have done, and control ministers who wanted to change the pattern of medical education in their provinces'.[139] The insistence of the Medical Council on the importance of 'practical training' in midwifery education including the personal supervision of twenty labour cases by each student evoked mixed reactions amongst medical men in different provinces. The Universities of Lucknow, Lahore and Burma responded by sending the fourth year students to the Government Maternity Hospital, Madras, for one month of training as intern students in order to provide them with facilities for observing obstetric operations and personally handling labour cases. In the case of Bengal, however, while the response of the Principal of the CMC and the other IMS officials was to placate the Council, the reaction of the indigenous medical men was more of a defensive and nationalistic nature.

Lieutenant Colonel F.A.F. Barnardo, Principal of the CMC, responded to the demands of the GMC by suggesting the establishment of an 'extern clinic'. He argued that the extern clinic would persuade more patients, mostly Anglo-Indian and poor women with little inhibitions, to avail themselves of attendance by male doctors. He also proposed three alternatives. In view of the intensive training in midwifery delivered in Bengal colleges for three years instead of one year in the British colleges, the Medical Council could be requested to accept six labour cases for individual training of students instead of the stipulated number of twenty. The second alternative could be to ask the Council to defer their decision to reject Indian degrees from February 1922 to February 1924. As a third option, he proposed the creation of a degree of the Bachelor of Obstetrics by the University of Calcutta which would be recognised by the Council.[140] The solution proposed by Bernardo reflected a conciliatory approach and also highlighted the fact that recognition by the Medical Council of Indian degrees was essential for the future of medical graduates in India.

On the other hand, the Bengali medical men's response was palpably of a defensive nature heavily tinged with nationalist sentiment.[141] M. N. Banerjee, the Principal of the Carmichael Medical College, defended the pedagogic infrastructure of the institution as one that was being constantly overhauled to meet the demands of the Medical Council and, hence, quite efficient. Also considering practical instructions to students in all labour cases as being adequate at the college, Banerjee commented that 'students are not allowed to attend cases – "somehow" as in extern maternities, neither are they allowed to attend cases merely to be "signed up" '.[142] Dr Kedarnath Das too retorted, stating clearly before the Annual Conference of the Indian Provincial Medical Services Association in 1921 that the medical education in India was quite adequate.[143] The Registrar of the Calcutta University, J. L. Ghosh, argued that the existing clinical materials at the disposal of the students and the tenure of three years for the teaching of midwifery were far better than many medical schools in the United Kingdom.[144] Previously, Kedarnath Das had challenged the statements and statistics of IMS officers who had submitted written statement to the Public Services Commission in 1913 about 'defective midwifery training'.[145]

The debate which crystallised around 'defective' midwifery training eventually led to a sense of yearning for independence from the strictures of colonial control over medical education in India. The editorial in the *Calcutta Medical Journal* commented:

> The supervision over the medical institutions in India is done by the University and recently by the Bengal Council of Medical Registration. Neither the Privy Council therefore, nor the General Council can have any direct authority over the Calcutta University in as much as the Calcutta University can exercise no authority over the institutions in the United Kingdom.[146]

In a similar vein, at the third All India Medical Conference held in Lahore on 28 December 1929, Dr Bidhan Chandra Roy condemned the decision of the Medical Council to appoint an inspector, asserting that

> We do not want an inspector sent by the GMC. But we desire the fullest enquiry by *ourselves* into the methods of teaching in the different universities . . . we want to raise ourselves in *our* own estimation and the world is bound to respect us in spite of the detractors.[147]

One of his professed goals was to develop 'medical education in *our own* way (emphasis mine)'.[148] In a similar vein, another prominent medical man condemned the craze for foreign degrees as a 'morbid expression of a slave mentality' and insisted on modifying the teaching of the Indian universities to suit international standards.[149] The nationalist resentment over GMC's action did not however stand in the way of medical colleges in Bengal making attempts to revitalise the structure of midwifery training by appointing more staff or getting the students to observe labour cases at the Calcutta Corporation–run maternity homes and the Visuddhananda Saraswati Marwari Hospital. GMC's control over the quality of medical education continued till the constitution of the Medical Council of India in 1933 that took over the task of maintaining uniform and decidedly high standards of university education in the country and ensuring that Indian degrees were recognised abroad.

## Conclusion

This chapter has outlined the various stages through which midwifery was institutionalised and transformed into a medical discipline in Bengal. Instead of uncritically assuming the centrality of female physicians in the process of medicalisation of childbirth, it has analysed the agency of male physicians not in terms of the extent of their accessibility to the upper-caste purdah women but in sustaining the structure of midwifery education and broadening the scope of surgical obstetrics in Bengal. In other words, the chapter has demonstrated that the contribution of male doctors was more at a discursive level than in the realm of actual practice.

In the decades following the GMC's withdrawal of recognition of Indian university degrees, the demand for medical *swaraj* (independence) consolidated. At the same time, the nationalist overtones of the indigenous medical men continued to resonate more strongly in the field of maternity and child welfare work. The next chapter will explain how medical professionals assumed the responsibility of popularising scientific midwifery that got entangled into a wider emotional debate on maternal and infant welfare in the nationalist era of the late colonial period.

## Notes

1 R.J. Kinkead, 'Obstetrics as a Branch of Education: Being an Address Introductory to the Course of Lectures in Obstetric Medicine in the Queen's College, Galway, for the Session 1878–79', *The British Medical Journal*, Vol.2, No.937, 1878, 870–871.
2 Ireland did not represent the highest standards of midwifery education in Britain in the nineteenth century. It was rather the medical doctorates of Edinburgh and Glasgow and the licences of their colleges of physicians and surgeons that represented the highest standard of medical education. London was also way behind Edinburgh. Yet Kinkead's views expressed at the Queen's University in Ireland reflect the changing perceptions of the British medical profession as a whole towards midwifery. While the

standard and quality of midwifery education varied across Ireland, Scotland and England, midwifery had acquired the status of medical science by mid-nineteenth century, a fact that was acknowledged in the whole of Britain and beyond.

3　Kinkead, 'Obstetrics as a Branch of Education', 871.

4　Irvine Loudon, *Death in Childbirth: An International Study of Maternal Care and Maternal Mortality, 1800–1950*, Oxford: Clarendon Press, 1992, see Chapter 12.

5　See for instance, Jean Donnison, *Midwives and Medical Men: A History of the Struggle for the Control of Childbirth*, London: Historical Publications Ltd, 1993; Jane B. Donegan, *Women and Men Midwives: Medicine, Morality and Misogyny in Early America*, New York: Greenwood, 1978; Charlotte G. Borst, *Catching Babies: The Professionalisation of Childbirth, 1870–1920*, Cambridge, MA: Harvard University Press, 1996; Lianne McTavish, *Childbirth and the Display of Authority in Early Modern France*, Aldershot: Ashgate, 2005.

6　Supriya Guha, 'A History of the Medicalisation of Childbirth in Bengal in the Late Nineteenth and Early Twentieth Centuries', Unpublished PhD dissertation, University of Calcutta, 1996; Dagmar Engels, 'The Politics of Childbirth: British and Bengali Women in Contest, 1890–1930', in *Beyond Purdah? Women in Bengal, 1890–1930*, New Delhi: Oxford University Press, 1996; Cecilia Van Hollen, *Birth on the Threshold: Childbirth and Modernity in South India*, New Delhi, Zubaan, 2003.

7　Shib Chunder Bose, *The Hindoos as They Are: A Description of the Manners, Customs and Inner Life of Hindoo Society in Bengal*, Second Edition, Calcutta: Thacker, Spink & Co., 1883, Prefatory note.

8　Bose's view should be accepted with caution. Being a Brahmo of the liberal reformist disposition, Bose might have taken a more critical view of the Hindu society and its cultural practices than might have existed in reality and hence, his agenda was chiefly a modernising one. His view is important in understanding the scepticism towards one's own society and culture that had come to dominate Bengali intellectual thought in the nineteenth century as a result of contact with Western civilisation.

9　Bose, *The Hindoos as They Are*, 22–25.

10　Ibid.

11　Lal Behary Dey, *Bengal Peasant Life*, London: Palgrave Macmillan, 1878, 38. Like Shib Chunder Bose, Lal Behary was a graduate of Scottish Church College who later converted to Christianity. Hence, Dey's views should also be accepted with some caution as it was essentially written from a reformist point of view.

12　For instance, a British medical professional described Bengali women's fear of surgery in the following words: 'It is however remarkable how very timid and reluctant they are to face bodily pain and to submit even to the smallest operation', Report of the Bengal Branch of the Countess of Dufferin Fund for the Year Ending, 30 November 1895, 6 as quoted in Chandrika Paul, 'The Uneasy Alliance: The Work of British and Bengali Medical Professionals in Bengal, 1870–1935', Unpublished PhD dissertation, University of Cincinnati, 1997, 297.

13　To cite an example, Dr Rufus C. Thomas, who was the chief medical officer in one of the princely states in the Northern part of India reminisced about the response of a husband whose wife had undergone caesarean section in 1934 in the following words: 'I had obtained the husband's permission to do a caesarean section, had actually removed the child, and was proceeding to suture the uterus, when the husband burst into the theatre and demanded to take his wife home immediately. When it was explained that the operation was almost over, he waited outside, and when I came out repeated his intention of taking her forthwith. The danger of such a course did not seem to impress him, though it was fully explained to him in his own language by my House Surgeon. After much argument, he eventually agreed to leave her in the hospital for a week. He made several nocturnal attempts to remove her before the week was up, and we finally had to let her go. Rufus C. Thomas, 'Some Surgical Difficulties in India', *The British Medical Journal*, Vol.1, No.3826, May 1934, 807.

14  See 'Midwifery in India', *Kai Tiaki*, October 1915, 192.

15  Margaret Balfour and Ruth Young, *The Work of Medical Women in India*, Oxford: Oxford university Press, 1929, 3.

16  Quoted in Christian Hochmuth, 'Patterns of Medical Culture in Colonial Bengal, 1835–1880', *Bulletin of the History of Medicine*, Vol.80, No.1, 2006, 51.

17  Maneesha Lal, 'The Politics of Gender and Medicine in Colonial India: The Countess of Dufferin Fund, 1885–1888,' *Bulletin of the History of Medicine*, Vol.68, No.1, Spring 1994, 29–66.

18  Dr Madhusudhan Gupta was initially a practitioner of Ayurveda or traditional Indian medicine. Later on he obtained training in western medicine and was in fact, the first Hindu to have dissected a human body and therefore, to have broken a long-standing religious taboo of the Indians against dissection. For details see Deepak Kumar, 'Medical Encounters in British India, 1820–1920', *Economic and Political Weekly*, Vol.32, No.4, January 1997, 166–170.

19  West Bengal State Archives (WBSA), *General Committee of the Fever Hospital and Municipal Improvements*, Miscellaneous Evidences and Papers, Appendix F, No.27, 1839, 87–88.

20  Ibid.

21  National Archives of India (NAI), GOI, Home Department, Public Branch, O.C, No.22, 1 September 1841.

22  Mel Gorman, 'Introduction of Western Science into Colonial India: Role of the CMC, *Proceedings of the American Philosophical Society*, Vol.128, No.2, September 1988, 276–298.

23  NAI, GOI, Home Department, Public Branch, O.C., Nos. 40/41, 24 March 1849.

24  Samita Sen and Anirban Das, 'A History of the Calcutta Medical College and Hospital, 1835–1936', in Uma Dasgupta, ed. *Science and Modern India*, New Delhi: Centre for Studies in Civilisations, 2011.

25  Ibid.

26  'The Calcutta Medical College', *Indian Medical Gazette*, Vol.1, 1 July 1866, 187.

27  WBSA, Proceedings of the Lieutenant Governor of Bengal, General Department, Medical Branch, Proceedings 1–7, August 1867.

28  Ibid.

29  Ibid.

30 Ibid.
31 Materia Medica is the Latin term for a body of knowledge about substances possessing therapeutic properties which are used for making medicines.
32 WBSA, General Department, Education Branch, Proceedings 8–11, 12–13, 18–22, February 1868.
33 Ibid.
34 'Native Midwifery', *The Indian Medial Gazette*, Vol.2, October 1868, 239.
35 David Arnold, *Colonising the Body: State Medicine and Epidemic Disease in Nineteenth-Century India*, Berkeley, Los Angeles and London: University of California Press, 1993.
36 Ibid.
37 For instance, Clara Swain was the first of such women missionaries who came from New York to Bareilly in the United Provinces on 8 November 1869 and was attached to the Women's Foreign Missionary Society of the Methodist Episcopal Church. Within few years, she had numerous patients, which led to the establishment of a dispensary in 1873 and a hospital in 1874 where Swain's patients were treated. Fanny Butler came to India in 1880 and was attached to the Church of Zenana Missionary Society in England. Butler worked in Jubbulpore and Bhagalpore. Others were Miss Hewlett who worked in Amritsar, Miss Rose Greenfield in Ludhiana, Miss Elizabeth Bielby in Lucknow and so on. See Balfour and Young, *The Work of Medical Women*, 16–25.
38 WBSA, General Department, Medical Branch, November 1871, Proceedings 38–43.
39 Ibid.
40 The resistance of the dhais to western methods of midwifery has already been noted by Balfour and Young. The recalcitrance of the dhais was also a major reason for the failure of the Victoria Memorial Scholarships Fund which was started in 1903 with the sole objective of training the dhais. Another problem was the lack of continued supervision of the dhais once they were trained. See Balfour and Young, *The Work of Medical Women*, 131–132.
41 Of late Sean Lang has argued in her study of maternity services in colonial Madras that, 'Madras Lying-In Hospital in fact played a prominent and pioneering role in maternity provision and midwifery training in India'. Lang further stated that, 'The quality of its state maternity provision proved a useful weapon for the Government of Madras in its long-running rivalry with the presidencies of Bombay and especially Bengal . . . The Government of Madras was particularly proud of its Lying-in Hospital'. For details, see Sean Lang, 'Drop the Demon Dai: Maternal Mortality and the State in Colonial Madras, 1840–1875', *Social History of Medicine*, Vol.18, No.3, 2005, 359 and 377–378.
42 WBSA, Municipal Department, Medical Branch, D.H. Collection, Proceedings 21–27, File No.3, 12 October 1881.
43 WBSA, Municipal Department, Medical Branch, Proceedings 2–5, January 1883.
44 The General Reports of the Public Instruction in Bengal recorded seven dhai candidates at the Eden Hospital in 1892, nine in 1895, eight in 1898

and seven in 1899. Cited in Fn20, in Geraldine Forbes, 'Education to Earn: Training Women in the Medical Professions', in Geraldine Forbes, ed. *Women in Colonial India: Essays on Politics, Medicine, and Historiography*, New Delhi: Chronicle Books, 2005.

45  WBSA, Judicial Department, Medical Branch, Proceedings 1–2, 5–6, October 1889.

46  Ibid.

47  'Maternal and Infant Mortality-II', *The Journal of the Association of the Medical Women in India*, Vol.V, No.II, August 1916, 20.

48  Balfour and Young, *The Work of Medical Women*.

49  Chitra Deb, *Mahila Daktar: Vin Groher Basinda*, Second Edition, Calcutta: Ananda Publishers, 2010.

50  Paul, 'The Uneasy Alliance'.

51  Mridula Ramanna, *Health Care in Bombay Presidency, 1896–1930*, Delhi: Primus Books, 2012, Introduction, 5.

52  Abala Das and Ellen D' Abreau eventually went to Madras Medical College to pursue a career in medicine due to the initial reluctance of the Calcutta Medical Council Authorities to open the gate of medical education to females. While Abala never practised medicine later, Ellen went on to pursue MB degree in 1887. See Geraldine Forbes, 'Medicine for Women: "Lady Doctors" in the Districts of Bengal', in Forbes, *Women in Colonial India*.

53  Balfour and Young, *The Work of Medical Women*, 103.

54  'Medical Education in Lower Bengal', *The Indian Medical Gazette*, Vol.20, March 1885, 77–78.

55  Paul, 'The Uneasy Alliance', 92.

56  Ibid.

57  Balfour and Young, *The Work of Medical Women*, 36.

58  'The Dufferin Fund', *The Indian Medical Gazette*, Vol.27, March 1892, 79.

59  'The Countess of Dufferin Fund', *The Indian Lancet*, Vol.7, 1 April 1896, 343. Geraldine Forbes' pioneering research reveals how some of them had longer careers than the IMS doctors. Some of them were Haimabati Sen in Hooghly district, Mussamut Idennessa in Mymensingh, Hemangini Devi at the Dufferin Hospital in Bankura, Menaka Devi at the Girish Chandra Hospital in Murshidabad, Priya Bala Guha in the Zuharunissa Female Hospital, Bogra etc. All of them were licentiate students between 1891 and 1894 at the Campbell Medical School. See fn29 *List of Qualified Medical Practitioners in Bengal 1903*, Calcutta: Bengal Secretariat Press, 1903, in Forbes, 'Medicine for Women', 130 and 96.

60  The newspaper *Sanjivani* was particularly vocal about its criticism of the Fund's discriminatory policies.

61  Forbes, 'Education to Earn', 112–116; Lal, 'The Politics of Gender and Medicine'.

62  'The Bengal Branch of the Countess of Dufferin's Fund', *The Indian Medical Gazette*, Vol.39, April 1904, 144.

63  Paul, 'The Uneasy Alliance', 92.

64  See Balfour and Young, *The Work of Medical Women*, 34–35; Supriya Guha, ' "The Best Swadeshi": Reproductive Health in Bengal, 1840–1940', in Sarah Hodges, ed. *Reproductive Health in India: History, Politics, Controversies*, Delhi: Orient Longman, 2006.

65 Chandrika Paul's detailed study of the Bengal Branch of the Dufferin Fund shows that the number of Hindu purdahnashin patients remained low till 1911 while number of Muslim patients steadily went up. See Paul, 'The Uneasy Alliance', 280.

66 The trend of hospitalisation had already accelerated within a decade of the foundation of the Fund. The Bengal branch of the Dufferin Fund report stated that 107,000 women were treated in Bengal in 1895 which was an increase over the previous year of about 27,000. It also referred to several new hospitals being built in the districts of Bengal. For details, see 'The Bengal Branch of the Dufferin Fund', *The Indian Lancet*, Vol.7, March 1896, 255. However, Chandrika Paul's detailed study showed the low attendance of Hindu middle-class women. See Paul, 'The Uneasy Alliance'.

67 'The Bengal Branch of the Countess of Dufferin's Fund', *The Indian Medical Gazette*, Vol.38, July 1903, 262–263.

68 Forbes, 'Medicine for Women'.

69 'Provisional Report on the Working of the Countess of Dufferin Fund', *The Journal of the Association of Medical Women of India*, Vol.1, No.4, November 1908, 8–12.

70 'Provisional Report on the Working of the Countess of Dufferin Fund', 8.

71 Balfour and Young, *The Work of Medical Women*, 45.

72 Report of the Bengal Branch of the Countess of Dufferin Fund for the Year ending 30 November 1896 quoted in Forbes, 'Medicine for Women', 137–138.

73 'Copy of Remarks Made by the Inspector-General of Civil Hospitals, Bengal, on the Lady Dufferin Victoria Hospital, Calcutta, on the 13 August 1910', *The Journal of the Association of Medical Women in India*, Vol.2, No.1, February 1911, 33–35.

74 Samiksha Sekhawat, 'Feminising Empire: The Association of Medical Women in India and the Campaign to Found a Women's Medical Service', *Social Scientist*, Vol.41, No.5/6, 2013, 65–81.

75 'Association of Medical Women in India and Its Fifty Years', *Journal of the Association of Medical Women in India*, Vol.XLV, No.4, November 1957, 111.

76 'Indian Medical Women', *The Journal of the Association of the Medical Women of India*, Vol.3, No.4, November 1911, 15.

77 'Association of Medical Women', 112.

78 Balfour and Young, *The Work of Medical Women*, 50.

79 For an elaborate understanding on the ways in which women doctors appropriated male professional ethos, see Ambalika Guha, 'The "Masculine" Female: Women Doctors in Colonial India, c.1870–1940', *Social Scientist*, Vol.44, Nos.5–6, May–June 2016, 49–64.

80 Nancy M. Theriot, 'Women's Voices in Nineteenth-Century Medical Discourse: A Step Towards Deconstructing Science', *Signs*, Vol.19, No.1, Autumn 1993, 1–31.

81 Regina Markell Morantz-Sanchez, *Sympathy and Science: Women Physicians in American Medicine*, New York and Oxford: Oxford University Press, 1985, 231.

82 Editorial, 'Medical Women and Present-Day Needs', *The Journal of the Association of the Medical Women in India*, Vol.25, No.4, November 1937, 43.

83  *All India Women's Conference*, Fourteenth Session, 62.

84  L.S. Mudaliar, 'Presidential Address', *Journal of the Indian Medical Association*, Vol.3, No.9, May 1934, 354–359.

85  'Gynaecological Congress: Calcutta Session-Dr Baman Das Mukherjee Elected Chairman of R.C.', *Amrita Bazar Patrika*, 12 March 1941.

86  N.A. Purandare, 'Presidential Address', in Subodh Mitra, ed. *Transactions of the Obstetric and Gynaecological Congress*, Calcutta, 1941, 31.

87  A slightly different version of this section has been published in the form of an article. For details, see Ambalika Guha, 'Beyond the Apparent: The Male Doctors and the Medicalisation of Childbirth in Bengal, 1840s-1940s', *Indian Historical Review*, Vol.44, No.1, June 2017, 1–18.

88  Monica H. Green, 'Gendering the History of Women's Healthcare', *Gender and History*, Vol.20, No.3, 2008, 487–518.

89  Here I use the term non-official journals to mean those journals which were published by indigenous medical men out of the ambit of government jurisdiction and financial support. *Calcutta Medical Journal* was the mouthpiece of the Calcutta Medical Club which was a professional but non-governmental organisation of Bengali doctors to promote the exchange of medical ideas and pursuit of research.

90  Guha, 'A History of the Medicalisation of Childbirth'.

91  W.R. Arney, *Power and the Profession of Obstetrics*, Chicago and London: Chicago University Press, 1982, 25.

92  Projit Bihari Mukharji, *Nationalising the Body: Medical Market, Print and Daktari Medicine*, London: Anthem Press, 2011, 85.

93  Mukharji, *Nationalising the Body*, 96–97.

94  I am not engaging with the trajectory of private practices of the *daktar*, my concern being solely confined to understanding the constitution of a medical discourse on childbirth in the vernacular medical print and the way new medical ideas shaped the perception of the general practitioners or *daktar*. Many of the students of the vernacular class of the Calcutta Medical College often engaged in private practice, serving the rich bhadralok of Calcutta. Private *daktari* practice in Bengal expanded from the 1880s. It was a result of the growth of private medical colleges providing medical education to those who could not make their way into the government medical colleges. While the government sought to regulate the activities of these *daktars* since the 1880s and eventually passed the Medical Registration Acts in 1913 and 1914, a handful of eminent Bengali physicians lauded the private daktars or *Haathurey* for providing medical treatment to the bulk of the Bengali population who could not afford to pay the fees of the qualified doctors. Mukharji, *Nationalising the Body*, 69.

95  Annada Charan Khastagir, *Manabjanmatattva, Dhatribidya, Nabaprasutosisu o Strijatirbyadhisangraha* (A Treatise on the Science and Practice of Midwifery with Diseases of Women and Children), Second Edition, Calcutta: Girish Vidyaratna, 1878.

96  Ibid.

97  Khirodaprasad Chattopadhyay, *Dhatribidya* (A Treatise on the Art of Midwifery), Calcutta: Oriental Press, 1886; Nagendranath Sengupta, *Sochitro Daktari Sikkha* (Medical Education with Pictorial Illustrations), Fourth Edition, Calcutta: Nagendra Printing Works, 1905.

98  Jadunath Gangopadhyay, '*Banglar Cikitsak Samaj* (The Medical World of Bengal)', *Cikitsa Sammilani*, Vol.6, April–June1889, 178–192.
99  '*Bhoomika* (Introduction)', *Cikitsa Prakasa*, Vol.1, No.1, April 1909.
100 Ibid.
101 J.H. Keeling, 'An Address on Modern Obstetrics', *The British Medical Journal*, Vol.2, No.1176, July 14, 1883, 59.
102 Editorial, 'The Address in the Section of Obstetrics and Gynaecology', *The British Medical Journal*, Vol.2, No.1916, September 18, 1897, 726–727.
103 Adrian Wilson opines in his extensive study of the rise of man-midwifery in England in the eighteenth century that there was an argument against surgical intervention and 'leaving the placenta to nature'. Such argument in favour of anti-interventionism was promulgated by the famous man-midwife William Hunter. Hunter, according to Wilson, had the privilege of overseeing and attending normal birth unlike the previous generation of man-midwives who could intervene with forceps only in case of complications requiring instrumental interference. For details, see Adrian Wilson, *The Making of Man-Midwifery: Childbirth in England, 1660–1770*, London: UCL Press, 1995, Chapter 13.
104 Licentiate in Medicine and Surgery (LMS) or Vernacular Licentiate in Medicine and Surgery (VLMS) were medical degrees conferred by the Calcutta University and other universities in British India. It was equivalent to the MB degree and of the same duration of five years but the curriculum of the latter (i.e. MB) was larger. The licentiate degree holders occupied subordinate positions in the government medical services.
105 John W. Byers, *Prasabante Shonit Sraab Nibaron Ebong tahar Cikitsa'Bishak Darpan*, Vol.10. No.10, October 1900, 417–429. This essay was a Bengali translation of John W. Byer's presentation at the 68th annual symposium of the British Medical Association in 1900.
106 Keeling, 'An Address on Modern Obstetrics', 58.
107 Pulinchandra Sanyal, '*Sutikar-Tarunjworba Prasutir Pochajwar* (Puerperal Septicemia)', *Cikitsa Sammilani*, Vol.5, 1889, 114–119 and 227–229.
108 Rameshchandra Roy, '*Prasutir Proti Kartabya* (Duty Towards a Parturient Women)', *Bishak Darpan*, Vol.15, No.11, November 1905, 423–425.
109 '*Sutikagriha*', *Antahpur*, Vol.5, No.7, 1903, 135; '*SwargataKusumkumari* (Late Kusumkumari)', *Mahila*, Vol.3, No.1, August 1897, 21–22.
110 Dr Nagendranath Roy, '*Cikitsito Rogir Biboron: Prasab Durghatana* (Description of a Patient Treated: Accidents in Labour)', *Cikitsa Prakasa*, Vol.7, No.3, July 1915, 346–352.
111 Abhaykumar Sarkar, *Prasutiparicharya o sisu palan* (Treatment of the Pregnant Woman and Infant Rearing), Calcutta: The Calcutta Publishers, 1937, 13.
112 Sarkar, *Prasutiparicharya*, 17.
113 Sarkar, *Prasutiparicharya*, 22–23.
114 Devendranath Roy, *Garhasthya Svasthyaraksha o sochitro dhatrisiksha* (Domestic Hygiene and Guide to Bengali Midwives), Calcutta: S.K. Lahiri & Co, 1904.
115 Similarly, Kalikinkar Bhattacharya's monograph on 'The Science of Obstetrics' written in Bengali was dedicated to the education of midwives

and female health visitors in the villages of Bengal. See Kalikinkar Bhattacharya, *Prasaba-Vijnana* (A Treatise on Obstetrics), Calcutta: U.N. Dhar & Co, 1936. Sundari Mohan Das, who was the professor of midwifery and the Principal of the 'Jatiya Ayurvigyan Vidyalaya', wrote an extensive tract on midwifery and infant welfare by omitting 'some discarded views' and substituting them with 'modern views'. Sundari Mohan Das, *Saral Dhatri-Siksa, Kumar Tantra o Stri-Rog* (A Treatise on Midwifery, Infant-Rearing and Female Diseases), Calcutta: Premananda Das and Jogananda Das, 1940, Preface.

116 Some of the tracts on the gynaecological ailments of women were for instance, Harinarayan Bandopadhyay, *Strirogbidhayak* (The Diseases of Women – Medical and Surgical – with Special Reference to Indian Diseases), Second Edition, Calcutta: The New Saraswati Press, 1896; Nityananda Sinha, *Saphala Stri Cikitsa* (A Treatise on the Treatment of Diseases of Women), Audulbaria: Dr Dhirendranath Halder, 1915; Kiranchandra Ghosh, *Stri-Cikitsa* (A Treatise on the Diseases of Women and Gynaecology), Calcutta: Kiranchandra Ghosh, 1922.

117 Radha Raman Biswas, *Garbhini o Prasuti Cikitsa* (Treatment of Pregnant Woman and Infant), Calcutta: Walker Homeo Hall, 1938. There were other homeopathic tracts like Mahendranath Ghosh, *Saudaminira Dhatrisiksa Evam Garbhini o Prasuti Cikitsa* (A Work on Midwifery and Homeopathic Gynaecology), Calcutta: The Author, 1909; Kisorimohan Ghosh, *Garbhini Cikitsa* (Homeopathic Treatment in Pregnancy), Deoghar: The Criterion, 1914.

118 For instance, Harimohan Dasgupta, *Ayurvediya Dhatrividya Samgraha* (A Compilation of Ayurvedic Midwifery), Berhampur: The Author, 1917. Also see Binod Bihari Rai, *Ayurved Mote Sisupalan* (Infant Rearing According to Ayurveda), Rajshahi: Binod Press, 1891.

119 See 'Dr Kedar Das No More: Great Obstetrician', *The Amrita Bazar Patrika*, 4 March 1936. Apart from Kedarnath Das, there were other eminent doctors as well who had made their mark in the sphere of obstetrics. For instance, Dr Satish Chandra De who had served as a Resident Surgeon at the Eden Hospital was a distinguished student of the CMC who went on to receive Goodeve scholarship and later on a gold medal for proficiency in midwifery. In fact, Dr Joubert, the Professor of Midwifery at Eden Hospital, testified to his abilities stating that De's practical work was good and that he had acquired considerable experience in midwifery and diseases of women. See 'Scarps and Comments: Babu Satish Chandra De, M.A., M.B.', *Amrita Bazar Patrika*, 29 June 1894, 7. Other renowned male obstetricians of the period who flourished in other parts of India at around the same time were Dr A.L. Mudaliar (Madras), Dr N.A. Purandare (Bombay), Dr V.N. Shirodkar (Bombay) etc. For details see Helaine Selin, *Encyclopaedia of the History of Science, Technology and Medicine in Non-Western Cultures*, The Netherlands: Kluwer Academic Publishers, Vol.1, 1997, 95–96.

120 'Sir Kedarnath Das, C.I.E., M.D', *The British Medical Journal*, April 1936, 670–671.

121 NAI, GOI, Home Department, Medical Branch, A, Proceedings 114, April 1900.

122 'Sir Kedarnath Das, C.I.E., M.D.'.

123 Kedarnath Das, *Obstetric Forceps: Its History and Evolution*, Calcutta: The Art Press, 1928, see the Prefatory Notes.

124 Kedarnath Das, 'The Bengal Forceps: A Modified Obstetric Forceps for Use in Bengali Women', *The Indian Medical Gazette*, Vol.55, January 1923.

125 Chuni Lal Mukherjee, 'The Place of Forceps in Obstetrics', *Calcutta Medical Journal*, Vol.36, No.5, November 1939, 316–333.

126 Bibhuti Bhushan Bhattacharya, 'The Future Obstetrical Forceps', *Calcutta Medical Journal*, Vol.19, No.3, September 1924, 110–115.

127 Mukherjee, 'The Place of Forceps', 333.

128 Kedarnath Das, 'Midwifery in India', *Indian Medical Record*, Vol.44, February 1924, 42.

129 Kedarnath Das, *A Handbook of Obstetrics for Students in India*, London: Butterworth, 1914; Kedarnath Das, *A Text Book of Midwifery for Medical Schools and Colleges in India*, Second Edition, Calcutta: Thacker, Spink & Co, 1926.

130 Scopolamine and morphine were a form of obstetric anaesthesia that was discovered in the wake of the discovery of surgical anaesthesia. The use of scopolamine and morphine was systematised by Dr Gauss under the supervision of Dr Kronig in Freiburg, Germany, in the first decade of the twentieth century. The condition was named as 'Dammerschalf' by Gauss. The English renaming of 'Dammerschalf' as 'twilight sleep' became more popular. For details see R.C.B., 'The Search for Painless Child Birth', *The British Medical Journal*, Vol.1, No.2842, June 1915, 1052–1053.

131 The Twilight Sleep experiment which relieved women of the pains of childbirth became popular with the middle-class women in America. Newspapers and magazines supported the middle-class women's cry for greater application of scopolamine in childbirth by the medical profession. It grew into a national movement. However, many American doctors opposed the use of scopolamine as 'pseudo-scientific rubbish' and as something capable of causing harm to the mother or child. For details, see Judith Walzer Leavitt, 'Birthing and Anaesthesia: The Debate Over Twilight Sleep', *Signs*, Vol.6, No.1, Autumn 1980, 147–164. In the Indian context, it's difficult to gauge the response of Indian or Bengali women to the 'twilight sleep' controversy of 1916 and 1917 as the feminist consciousness had not yet consolidated on an organisational level prior to the 1920s.

132 J.M. Das, 'Scopolamine and Morphine Narcosis in Child-Birth', *The Calcutta Medical Journal*, Vol.15, No. 1, November 1918, 53. Other prominent obstetricians like V.B. Green-Armytage also supported the use of Twilight Sleep and were claimed to have achieved 'excellent results'. For details also see Cecil Webb Johnson, 'A Plea for Painless Childbirth in India', *The Indian Medical Gazette*, Vol.52, September 1917, 311–312.

133 'Council Proceedings: Official Report', *Bengal Legislative Council*, Forty-Ninth Session 1936, Alipore, Bengal: Bengal Government Press, 1936.

134 J.M. Das, 'Obstetric Impression', *The Indian Medical Gazette*, Vol.55, 1923.

135 Ibid.

136  V.B. Green-Armytage, 'A Plea for the Lower Uterine Segment Caesarean Section', *The Indian Medical Gazette*, Vol.66, April 1931. V.B. Armytage also authored an extremely important book entitled '*A Textbook of Midwifery in the Tropics*' which was considered a product of his long experience as the professor of midwifery which 'fitted him to write a book dealing with midwifery as modified by racial and climatic conditions . . . and gauge the value of those lines of treatment most applicable to the East, particularly India'. See 'Book Review', *Indian Medical Gazette*, Vol.68, March 1933, 174.

137  M.V. Webb, 'Surgical Intervention in Obstetric Practice', *The Journal of the Association of the Medical Women of India*, Vol.25, No.4, November 1937, 5–10.

138  WBSA, Government of Bengal, Local Self Government, Medical Branch, Proceedings 21–48, File 2M-13, December 1926.

139  Roger Jeffery, *The Politics of Health in India*, Berkeley and Los Angeles: University of California Press, 1988, 85.

140  WBSA, Government of Bengal, Local Self-Government Department, Medical Branch, Progs. 7–22, File 3M-3, June 1922.

141  It is relevant to mention here an incident that was reported in the nationalist press in 1909; the incident reflected the dissatisfaction of the Bengalis with the allegedly faulty way of conducting midwifery examination at the CMC. It was ruefully reported that of the fifty-three candidates at the Medical College, forty-five failed due to their unsuccessful performance in midwifery. This implied a loss of one full year as the students would not be allowed to sit for the examination which was scheduled to be held after six months. The failure of the students was ascribed to the faulty way of conducting the oral exam and not to the poor performance of the students themselves. It was alleged that during the oral exam three hours for eight students were allotted to Medicine, four hours for twelve students to Surgery while only forty-five minutes for eight students was given to midwifery. This erratic and arbitrary method of examining the students was considered as 'wholesale slaughter' at the final examination. This incident reflects the disgruntlement of the Bengalis with the government's tendencies to marginalise midwifery even when there was no dearth of brilliant students around. See, *The Amrita Bazar Patrika*, 9 June 1909, 7.

142  Ibid.

143  'Problem of Midwifery Training in Indian Medical Colleges', *Calcutta Medical Journal*, Vol.19, No.4, October 1924, 160.

144  WBSA, Government of Bengal, Local Self-Government Department, Medical Branch, Proceedings 7–22, File 3M-3, June 1922.

145  'Problem of Midwifery Training', 158.

146  'Editorial', *Calcutta Medical Journal*, Vol.19, No.3, September 1924, 131.

147  'Medical News: All India Medical Conference', *Calcutta Medical Journal*, Vol.24, No.7, January 1930, 302.

148  Ibid.

149  A.C. Ukil, 'The Teaching of Medicine in the Calcutta University', *The Calcutta Medical Journal*, Vol.XIX, No.4, October 1924, 148.

# 3 Maternal and child welfare

## A nationalist concern in late colonial Bengal, 1900–1940s

From the second decade of the twentieth century, a section of the Bengali intelligentsia including the medical professionals and women activists became enthusiastic participants in the global discourse on child welfare movement. All the same, the exasperations over loss of infant and maternal life were effectively linked to the furore over the future of the budding Indian nation in a way that invested the issue with an immediacy and potency that had not existed before.

In an essay submitted to the Madras press in 1927 Dr Muthulakshmi Reddy, an eminent local woman physician, pithily summed up the significance of the child welfare movement by basing it on her first-hand experience of the movement in European countries in the 1920s. She stated:

> Child-welfare work is of such a wide national concern that it ought to interest not only the proper health authorities and the medical profession, but also the State, the statesman, the patriot and the lay-public, because the child of today is the patriot of tomorrow. If we want our future generation of young men to command a robust physique and a healthy intellect, the health training ought to commence even from the very beginning of life, from the movement of the conception in the mother's womb.[1]

This chapter explores how the maternal and infant welfare discourse that acquired prominence in Bengal in the interwar years provided ideological justification for bringing pregnancy and childbirth under medical supervision in order to fulfil the broader nationalist objective of promoting the healthy growth of the nation. It argues that the dual engagement of Bengali medical professionals with the nationalist rhetoric of motherhood and the global eugenic concern for better racial stock provided the rationale for 'expert medical control, developing, co-ordinating and directing all effort, voluntary and official, towards the one common goal of robust individual health and racial improvement'.[2] Preserving the life of the expectant mother and the child as the basis of a healthy nation was reckoned as the most pressing logic for the 'medical men and women' to 'share the burden as a joint responsibility' and to organise themselves and 'combine to uplift the condition of the expectant mothers' and also to 'educate our friends, and neighbours about the necessity of their womenfolk and children being examined by doctors'.[3]

The origin of the infant welfare movement as an organised and systematic movement in western countries is usually traced to the years following the First World War. From the end of the nineteenth century, the declining birth rate began to provoke public interest in the need to prevent wastage of infant life in England and other European countries. This led to medical probes into the causes of infant mortality and resulted in investigative research being conducted by eminent medical men like Dr Longstaff in 1880, Dr Ballard in 1887 and Dr Newsholme in 1889. As both Jane Lewis and Anna Davin have argued, the massive loss of life during the Anglo-South African (Boer) War (1899–1902) triggered grave concerns about the deteriorating national standards of physical health. Infant welfare conferences were held in Paris (1905), Brussels (1907), London (1908) and Berlin (1911). In England laws were passed in the hope of improving conditions of childbirth including the Midwives Act of 1902 and the Children's Act of 1908. Voluntary societies such as Infants' Health Society (1904), the National League for Health, Maternity and Child Welfare (1905), Eugenics Education Society (1908) etc. sprang up for promoting public health awareness amongst the masses.[4] Equally significant was the intervention of municipal authorities in launching cheap milk supply schemes and organising conferences on infant mortality in 1906 and 1908. However, it was the outbreak of the First World War (1914–18) that sharpened public anxieties about the devastating impact of the loss of human lives on the national health. The consequence, as G. F. McCleary argued, was

> the uprising of the national spirit which sought expression in various kinds of activity for the national good. To many it seemed that caring for the mothers and babies of the country was work of special importance at that time – a form of war-work that called for the enlistment of many workers.[5]

In the post-1918 years, preserving the health of infants in ensuring the healthy growth of the population and improving the racial stock was paralleled by efforts to reduce maternal mortality.

Reverberations of the infant welfare movement were felt across the globe. India, being one of the strongholds of British Empire, came to appropriate concerns for maternal and infant health in a way that helped forge its own sociopolitical agendas of nationhood. The chapter will demonstrate how debates on the importance of maternal and infant life came to reflect nationalist imperatives of the Bengalis in the post-Swadeshi era.[6] The socio-economic factors causing infant and maternal mortality in Bengal such as child marriage, early maternity, poverty and lack of adequate milk supply were amply recognised in the nationalist press and in the writings of Bengali medical men. Yet the solution was sought not so much in directly addressing the socio-economic issues as in advocating medicalisation of childbirth and professional supervision of pregnancy and infant health.

The public health policies in Bengal which were hitherto confined to regulating sanitary measures and addressing epidemic diseases such as malaria, cholera, influenza, *Kala-Azar* etc. were expanded in the twentieth century to include maternal and child welfare schemes. From 1908 onwards, local bodies in Calcutta, mainly the Calcutta Corporation, initiated health visiting schemes that, by 1914, were tied to the objective of combating infant mortality caused by tetanus neonatorum. From the second decade of the twentieth century, maternal and infant health was gradually incorporated as an integral component of public health policies, as it was in England and elsewhere.[7] It signalled a more comprehensive role for the public health workers and medical professionals requiring them to analyse the health conditions of expectant mothers in their specific socio-economic settings. It also entailed educative and health awareness schemes for the lay public that included exhibitions, baby shows and lectures with the aid of magic lantern slides and documentary films.[8] The redefined public health administration shaped the contours of maternity and infant care services in Calcutta and the outlying districts in Bengal.

The chapter is divided into two main sections: the first section will trace the constitution of a medical discourse on maternal and infant health that was heavily laced with social, nationalistic and eugenic concerns in the interwar years. Drawing upon Jane Lewis's argument on how maternal and infant mortality was defined chiefly in terms of a series of medical problems in England,[9] the chapter will demonstrate how the Bengali medical men, both obstetricians and licentiate doctors, seized upon the public concerns for maternal and infant health in order to assert the need for greater medical control and professional supervision over pregnancy and childbirth. Reforming the conditions of childbirth was at the same time driven by the highly emotionalised rhetoric of motherhood that prodded the medical profession to articulate its role in nationalist terms. At the Second All India Obstetrics and Gynaecological Congress held in Bombay in 1937 the renowned Bengali obstetrician Bamandas Mukherjee claimed that, 'what we should all bear in mind is, that in any future plan of national reconstruction, outlined by the State, the Obstetrician and the Gynaecologist will have a very important role to perform'.[10] The essence of an obstetrician's work, according to Mukherjee, lay in adopting suitable educational measures and propaganda work to eradicate maternal ignorance and rescue Indian mothers from the clutches of untrained dhais. Coordination between the government, the medical profession and an 'enlightened' public was perceived as being central to the nation-building work.[11]

The second part of this chapter will critically evaluate the implementation of maternal and child welfare schemes in Bengal by focusing particularly on the role of local bodies like the Calcutta Municipal Corporation and newly evolved institutions like the All India Institute of Hygiene and Public Health in extending the scope of maternity services to a larger section of the population consisting mainly of the lower middle class and the slum dwellers in Calcutta. Drawing upon the annual reports of the Calcutta Corporation and the Public Health Department, it will argue that the contribution of the Calcutta Municipal Corporation was pivotal to the expansion of modern maternity services, in creating new categories of health visitors and domiciliary midwives and also in promoting the shift of the site of birth from home to hospitals and maternity homes under its auspices. Much of it was, however, an emulation of maternal and child welfare work in England in the interwar years.

## Mother of the nation

The relevance of maternal and infant health in the broader nationalist vision was far from being clearly spelt out in the late nineteenth century. The bhadralok's concerns for physical health of the Bengalis sometimes led to recognition of certain social customs as being responsible for the declining health of mothers and the birth of weak infants. Such arguments were usually framed by medical men of the bhadralok class with professedly dual commitments towards social reforms and the advancement of western scientific medicine. Towards the end of the nineteenth century, the medical men started a number of health journals in Bengali language with the goal of spreading health education amongst the masses. Dissemination of scientific–medical explanations of pregnancy and management of maternal and infant health in familiar cultural and nationalist terms constituted one of the chief functions of such journals. Such journals are to be distinguished from medical journals such as *Bishak Darpan* and *Cikitsa Prakasa* that contained matters of academic interest directly related to the expansion of professional knowledge and, hence, meant chiefly for professional readership.

Concerns for 'national health' (*jatiya Svasthya*) found increasing expression in the popular print from the last two decades of the nineteenth century. In 1885 *Cikitsa Sammilani* complained that the 'Bengalis, who are too easily moved by the apparent importance of issues, fail to see the real Bengali issue of improving their physical health'.[12] The long-standing idea of physical weakness came to be associated with racial degeneracy (*jatikkhoy*). The solution envisaged in such journals was two-fold: an engagement with the notion of enlightened motherhood as the key to rearing healthy citizens. At the same time, the responsibility of preserving maternal health as crucial for curtailing infant mortality and ensuring the birth of healthy infants was also underscored. Second, the urgency of recognising child marriage as a potent societal evil causing early maternity (untimely pregnancies) and the birth of weak infants was driven home. Child marriage and early maternity were increasingly addressed and explained through the prism of eugenics.

The trope of motherhood was particularly powerful in Bengal. While mothers' social responsibility in rearing healthy and morally upright children for the prospective Indian nation was emphasised in the nationalist discourse from the early twentieth century, maternal ignorance was touted as a major stumbling block causing sickness and mortality amongst infants. The rhetoric of motherhood in Bengal had historical roots in the portrayal of nation as mother in Bankim Chandra Chattopadhyay's proto-nationalist novel *Anandamath* published in 1878. Abanindranath Tagore's painting of '*Bharat Mata* (Mother India)' further added a strong patriotic dimension to the nationalist imagery of motherhood during the Swadeshi era (1903–08).[13] According to Jasodhara Bagchi, what set Bengal apart from other regions of India was 'the prevalence of goddess worship' which 'certainly facilitated the empowering of the mother-image in Bengal so that it becomes the most dominant myth of colonial Bengal'.[14] Bengal's long-standing tradition of worshipping Shakti, Kali, Durga and Savitri – the various mythological forms of mother goddess – had resonances in the bhadralok imagination of the nation as a feminine entity.

Margaret M. Urquhart's pioneering ethnographic research on the purdahnashin Bengali women in the 1920s traced the worship of mother goddess in Bengal to the sacrosanct and intense relationship between the mother and her son. To quote Urquhart,

> Love of her son is the ruling passion of the Bengali woman, at least so it would appear to the onlooker . . . It is, perhaps, the intensity of this relation that has influenced Hindu religious thought and expression so profoundly. To the Hindu it is the mother aspect of God that calls for his most fervent worship.[15]

Recent historical and anthropological researches on Bengali women confirm Urquhart's views on the nuances of mother–son relationship in Bengal. According to Bharati Ray, mother–son 'emotional bond' was more powerful than any other relationship constituting the 'core' of the mother's 'uterine family'.[16] Manisha Roy's anthropological study of Bengali women in the 1960s and 1970s further shed light on the intense bonding between the mother and a son, seeking its roots in the customs of the son sleeping close to mother, familial codes forbidding physical and emotional attachment with father and, lastly, the practice of late weaning.[17]

Urquhart's study brought to the fore the centrality of mother's role within the family. The mother was envisioned as the model of rectitude, and as an essay entitled *Adarsha Janani* (Ideal Mother) stated, 'the symbol of order, peace and prosperity in the household. She serves everyone and epitomises the splendour and beauty of the loving goddess . . . the mother should cultivate the spiritual qualities of broadmindedness, affection, softness of heart, simplicity, tolerance and kindness'.[18] The religious connotations attached to motherhood came out more sharply in another article published in *Bamabodhini Patrika* in 1886 in which love for mother was equated with devotion to god. It called for absolute dedication of the son to his mother in his craving for peace, knowledge and love.[19]

In the post-Swadeshi era, the role of the mother was reconceptualised in terms of her paramount contribution to the nation-building activities by creating and nurturing a strong race. As Sumit Sarkar has pointed out, Swadeshi movement in Bengal contributed, in myriad ways, towards shaping the trend of nationalist politics till the end of colonial rule.[20] The nation-building activities in the post-Swadeshi phase constituted a step-by-step revitalisation of national life including reviving 'autonomous' economy, education, family and health. In this milieu the nation-building aspect of a mother's role was repeatedly asserted in prescriptive pamphlets such as *Adarsha Janani* or ideal mother (1914), *Santan Palan* or childrearing (1915), *Sisu Palan* or infant rearing (1916) and *Jananir Prati* or address to the mother (1919).[21]

Despite the role of mother being redefined in national terms, maternal ignorance was trolled in the media as a major factor affecting mortality rates from the early decades of the twentieth century. In England, as Anna Davin has argued, maternal ignorance was cited as the most important factor for explaining rising infant mortality at the cost of marginalising other factors such as medical ignorance, poverty and lack of access to medical care.[22] In Bengal maternal ignorance was, however, not the central point of criticism although it did come to be recognised as a dominant factor causing infant mortality along with poverty, poor hygiene and ignorance of the dhais.

To offer an example, Ramesh Chandra Ray, a licentiate doctor, undertook a systematic survey of the conditions of the Bengali school boys in April 1916. Finding the 'poor physique, the feminine build and carriage . . . of our school boys' Ray went on to investigate the causes of infant mortality and weak physique of the children. Of all the causes highlighted such as lack of nourishment of the mother, insanitary conditions of Bengali homes or attack of malaria during pregnancy, maternal ignorance was cited as one of the prime factors. It was argued that an average Bengali girl had

> no knowledge of the immense importance of breast-feeding, of the delicate mechanisms of the child's body and of the intricate functions of her own sex organs . . . This dense ignorance is responsible for the horrors of the Indian natal chamber as well as for all the evils wrought by the quack midwife in the name of self-advertised experience and efficiency.[23]

The remedy according to Ray lay in systematic training of girls and expectant mothers in mother-craft, a term borrowed from England.[24]

The subjects of mother-craft and housewifery were not new in Bengal, having roots in the late nineteenth-century reformist discourse. They were, however, freshly framed as matters of national interest in the interwar years. Mother-craft included training in subjects like physiology, hygiene, first aid, infant care, home nursing, diseases of the infants and their prevention and a general idea of maternity. In the years following the First World War, housewifery and mother-craft were beginning to be considered as integral to a woman's contribution to society and towards saving 'the soul of the future nation'.[25] However, Samita Sen's research on working-class women in the Bengal jute mills reveals class differences being ignored in the application of such thoroughly middle-class notions of mother-craft to the poor working-class women. As Sen argues, the compulsion of working-class mothers to earn outside home in order to feed their children and the consequent responsibility of the children to manage household work led to dominant middle-class notions of motherhood being undermined.[26] The discussion on motherhood was not solely confined to delineating women's role in rearing the future citizens of the nation. Conditions of maternal health also came increasingly under medical scrutiny and became the subject of intense public discussion in the early twentieth century.

## Early maternity and the dying Hindu race

The question of infant and maternal mortality assumed national importance in the aftermath of the Swadeshi movement in Bengal, evoking divergent responses from the nationalists and the British officials.[27] The British officials and western observers squarely blamed the 'moribund' Bengali social customs of child marriage, and 'bad midwifery' for infant and maternal mortality. The census reports and annual reports of the Calcutta Municipal Corporation and Public Health Department documented the 'official' view. The Census of 1911, for instance, attributed high infant mortality to 'premature birth', 'debility at birth', 'bad midwifery' and 'tetanus neonatorum due to the umbilical cord being cut with dirty instruments'.[28] In 1914, H. M. Crake, the Health Officer of the Calcutta Corporation, identified similar causes further linking 'tetanus neonatorum' to 'ignorance and defective midwifery practices' and attributing 'debility at birth' and 'premature birth' to 'the economic and social conditions of the people, particularly poverty, insanitary conditions, child marriage and the purdah, a baffling group of causes'.[29] During a Legislative Council debate, the Bengal Government clearly refrained from taking any 'special action' to reduce the high proportion of infant deaths, arguing that the deaths had a lot to do with the 'domestic life and social customs' of the Bengalis and hence could not be eradicated easily.[30] While economic conditions and poverty of the masses were recognised as obstacles, they were certainly not considered as the most significant factors causing infant and maternal deaths.

The nationalists were more disposed towards critiquing the economic policies of the state, lack of pure milk supply and bad housing conditions in Bengal than accepting *prima facie* the colonial invective on Bengali sociocultural practices.[31] In this connection, the Bengali health magazine *Svasthya Samachar* pointed out that 'if social customs were the main reasons behind infant mortality, both the communities (Hindu and Muslim) would have ceased to exist long back'.[32] The nationalist press critically observed that the government had done little beyond suggesting few elementary measures such as the appointment of municipal midwives, although such suggestions were invariably followed by 'plentiful doses of gratuitous sermons on the ignorance and apathy of people themselves'.[33]

Nationalist response was seldom homogeneous swerving uncomfortably from being defensive and traditionalist (as evident during the Age of Consent Bill Controversy when child marriage and early consummation were defended on religious and traditional grounds) to being self-critical, secular and modernist (as in the interwar years). For instance, the aspersions cast on the traditional dhais were a common factor in colonial and nationalist attitude and, hence, constituted a form of self-criticism by the nationalists. With an equal ardour the time-honoured custom of child marriage was denounced from the second decade of the twentieth century. Notwithstanding the massive conservative uproar over the Age of Consent Bill (1891) that raised the age of sexual consummation for girls from ten to twelve, public opinion continued to be divided on the wisdom behind preserving the custom of child marriage. In the interwar years however, child marriage was unequivocally condemned in the enlightened middle-class discourses reflecting eugenic concerns of the Bengalis for the decline of the nation.

At the turn of the century, arguments about the weak constitution of the Bengalis were being emphatically tied to the social practices of child marriage, multiple marriage, alcoholism and masturbation. However, it was in the condemnation of child marriage that the eugenic sensibilities of the Bengalis became most conspicuous. As Sarah Hodges has argued, marriage reforms were central to the eugenics discourse in India, meagre attention being otherwise paid to eugenics research and investigations into the specific mechanisms of heredity. The focus of Indian eugenicists was, exclusively on caste-based 'arranged marriages' with purported roots in ancient Indian society. Arranged marriages were perceived as the quintessential Indian way of uniting couples capable of producing healthy offspring. As part of the eugenics discourse, reform of child marriage was connected to reproductive health and national progress,[34]

Reflecting upon how child marriage was related to questions of health, an essay published in 1901 in *Svasthya* argued:

> It is usually seen that children of healthy parents are strong and healthy, whereas weak children result from a marriage between parents in poor health . . . it needs no great effort to show that the primary reason for the weak constitution of Bengalis lies in the custom of child marriage practised by them.[35]

While lack of nutritious food and physical exercise were also recognised as major factors, child marriage was considered as a 'far more important' factor in producing weak and unhealthy children. U. N. Mukherji's book entitled *Hindus – A Dying Race* published in 1909 seized upon such anxieties to portray morbid picture of a shrivelling, physically weak Hindu race as opposed to a strong and blooming Muslim population.[36] Mukherji's central idea of the extinction of the Hindus heavily impinged upon the consolidation of a communal ideology in Bengal.[37] The imagery of a 'dying Hindu race' had strong resonances in the writings of medical men and educated middle-class women, particularly in their apprehensions about the diminishing vitality of the nation. Thus, in 1919, the prominent women's magazine *Bharati* considered child marriage and early maternity leading to maternal mortality as the chief factors facilitating the decline in national health and deterioration of race.[38]

A distinct eugenic argument was also visible in writings that reflected an interest in preserving purity of the Bengalis through preventing marriages between unfit partners. For instance, in an interesting article entitled *Bibahopon o Svasthya* ('Dowry and Health') published in 1901, linkages were drawn between women's health and the deeply entrenched social custom of dowry. It was alleged that the greed of the guardians negotiating profitable marriage deals often blinded them to any 'genetic disease' running in the family or the possibilities of ailments like rheumatism, tuberculosis, asthma and contagious diseases being passed on to the offspring.[39] The example of dowry was one of the ploys evolved by the bhadralok medical men in explaining the role of an 'inappropriate marriage' in accentuating the chances of 'genetic diseases' being transmitted from parents to children.

Anxieties over 'congenital defects' of parents and their impact on racial vitality of the nation intensified in the changed political climate of the post-First World War years when maternal and infant health became global concerns. The pressure from post-war international bodies like the International Labour Organisation and the League of Nations sharpened the focus on the socioeconomic conditions in which birth took place. Comparative studies conducted by the League of Nations on factors affecting infant mortality in European and South American countries revealed congenital and developmental defects as potent causes of infant death.[40] Bengali health journals cautioned women on the need to be aware of those mental and physical disabilities of the infant which were induced by a combination of societal ills like child marriage and congenital diseases of parents. There were repeated warnings against the possibilities of venereal diseases like syphilis and gonorrhoea being directly transmitted to the offspring. Dr Ramesh Chandra Ray stated in 1919:

> Now that the subject of eugenics is so well known, it would be useless to note of time and space to dilate on the supreme necessity for choosing as life's partner one who is healthy in every sense of the term . . . if the State has the right to punish any individual who propagates disease, has it not the right to punish anyone who offers his syphilitic boy or girl in marriage?[41]

The Bengali medical men went to the extent of advising sickly individuals or those suffering from tuberculosis to abstain from getting married or having children.[42]

With the rise of Gandhian nationalism in the 1920s and the culture of mass politics it fostered, the predominance of Hindu cultural nationalism in Indian politics receded to the background. Gandhian movements encouraged participation of women in the public sphere as a form of devotional service to the nation. In such a milieu, the long-running controversies on child marriage and the sexual practices of the Indians acquired a nationalist–political hue with the publication of Katherine Mayo's *Mother India* in 1927. *Mother India* located the root of India's political immaturity and unfitness for self-rule in the Indian male's manner 'of getting into this world and his sex-life thereafter'.[43] Of all the vices mentioned early consummation and early maternity were particularly attacked and condemned. *Mother India*'s publication brought the connected themes of child marriage, maternal and infant mortality and eugenics to the forefront of fervent public debates. The protagonists in the debate interestingly included political leaders, social reformers, doctors, feminists and members of the ordinary public.

On the official side, an enquiry committee known as the Joshi Committee (the other name being Age of Consent Committee) was appointed in 1927 to investigate the actual nature of conjugal practices of the Indians. A pronounced eugenic sensibility ran through its conclusion: 'Early maternity is an evil and an evil of great magnitude. It contributes very largely to maternal and infantile mortality, in many cases wrecks the physical system of the girl and generally leads to degeneracy of the physique of the race'.[44] The Committee also concluded that not only early maternity, but also the frequency of births at short intervals coupled with the conditions under which birth took place had a strong bearing on maternal and infant health. Thus, Mayo's *Mother India*, despite being trenchantly criticised by virtually all sections of Indian society, triggered a vigorous campaign for eradicating the custom of child marriage. This time it met with greater success than before and led to the promulgation in 1929 of the Child Marriage Restraint Act (popularly known as the Sarda Act) which raised the marriageable age for girls to 14 and for boys to 18.

In the interwar years, one of the perceptible trends in the health journals was the manner in which 'national' health was defined in terms of drawing examples from other parts of the world. Nationalism was envisioned as a comprehensive development of the nation along modern/scientific lines in the global hierarchy of civilisations. Exemplary tales of advancements in maternal and child welfare work in European countries, America and New Zealand were published in popular health and women's magazines with a view to drawing middle-class readers into a cosmopolitanism that would facilitate the assimilation of international ideas into the nationalist discourse. It served to underscore the inabilities of the Bengalis and the Indian nation in grappling with the challenges of maternal and child mortality. The problems of overpopulation, illiteracy of women and the social customs of child marriage and early maternity were repeatedly cited as major barriers for advancing the cause of infant welfare in Bengal.[45]

Thus, the emerging discourse on maternal and infant welfare in Bengal was essentially brought into shape by the medical profession and diffused through the pages of popular health magazines. Discussions on maternal ignorance, child marriage and early maternity had already been in vogue from the end of the nineteenth century. However, they acquired a pronounced 'eugenic' overtone in the twentieth century, more so, in the post-1918 years. Pressure from international organisations and the flutter caused by the publication of Mayo's *Mother India* were equally powerful stimulants. The solution was sought in medical

remedies by the obstetricians, the public health officials, the nationalists and the educated middle-class women. It was thus not so much a
denial of socio-economic factors as an increased advocacy of medical
solutions that triggered the need for expanding the scope of maternity
services.

## Maternal and infant welfare work in the post-1918 years

In Bengal the initial maternal and infant welfare schemes implemented
in the post-1918 years were not nationalist endeavours per se. Instead
they were ventures undertaken by the vicereines thus indicating multiple drivers of change. The momentum was provided by the formation
of the National Health and Baby Week Council in England in 1917.[46]
The baby week and the infant welfare and health exhibition associated
with it were intended to create favourable atmosphere 'for an all-sided
study and consideration of this important National problem and thus
the public opinion so enlivened, can be taken advantage of in starting
permanent institutions like Health Associations'.[47] However, unlike
the situation in England, state intervention in India was limited, direct
state involvement being largely absent. It was mostly in the nature of
sanctioning semi-official enterprises which, in most cases, relied on
public subscription. The Association for the Provision of Health Visitors and Maternity Supervisors, founded in Delhi in 1918, is a case in
point.

The Association was the first serious effort to directly address the
issue of maternal and infant welfare in India. Its objective was to
remove

> the adverse conditions which too often attend child-birth in India
> and to educate and enlighten the people in those matters in which
> care is essential if the population of the country is to be conserved
> and the rising generations are to grow up as strong and healthy
> citizens . . . it is the object of the Association to . . . improve the
> knowledge and the work of dais.[48]

Thus, the Association aimed for improving the work of the dhais
rather than supplanting them altogether. Although the Association
was initially started with a grant of Rs 6,000 provided by the Government of India, the scheme ultimately had to rely on public subscription from the princes and chiefs of India. A similar health school came
into being in Calcutta in the 1920s through the initiative of the Red

Cross Society although its success in attracting candidates for training in health visiting was rather limited.[49]

The next milestone in the child welfare movement in India was the maternal and child welfare exhibition held in Delhi in 1920. Margaret Balfour ascribed the origin of the idea for the exhibition to the interest of Vicereine Chelmsford in the welfare of the women and children of India. According to Balfour, it was the Vicereine's relentless appeal for philanthropic contribution to the cause of child welfare work that the Lady Chelmsford League for Maternity and Child Welfare was founded in 1919. The exhibition was eventually held under the banner of the League.[50] It intended to conduct practical demonstrations about the harmful consequences of carelessness during childbirth by deploying models, pictures, lectures etc. in order to ensure greater intelligibility by the masses. The conviction underlying such efforts was that

> such exhibitions are of great value in stimulating public interest . . . The Exhibition may therefore be regarded as a useful supplement to the work of the Association and it is hoped that it may emphatically draw public attention to the value of the ends which the Association has in view.[51]

The Association set the trend in India for maternity and child welfare exhibitions which were, in the following years, conducted in different major cities and in the process, acquired a pan-Indian hue. Following its success, Vicereine Reading started the National Baby Week in 1924 highlighting the urgency of such events in the national life of the people. The concept of baby week was welcomed by a section of the Indian leaders and elites. One of them, the Begum of Bhopal, stated: 'The holding of an annual Baby Week is a great step forward in the direction to which energies must be spent if we wish to equip our women for the sacred duty of bringing up strong and healthy children who will stand the wear and tear of strenuous times ahead and be a source of pride to their race.'[52] Its importance also lay in turning the attention of the Indian public towards adopting a more comprehensive programme for remedying the ills of infant mortality at an educational, preventive, economic and social level.

In Bengal, 'Baby Shows' became part of the activities of the Dufferin Hospitals.[53] The nationalists' response towards the practical utility of such 'western' propaganda methods in arousing the interest of middle-class women was initially sceptical. Proposals to educate the fathers and husbands who were thought to be responsible for the well-being of the mother and the newborn infant were floated as more viable alternatives.[54] Such western propaganda methods appeared less alien and more Indian with the intervention of Bengali middle-class women from the 1920s.

## Maternal and child welfare and the women's organisations

From the 1920s, Bengali middle-class women directly embraced midwifery work. Utilising the platform of *mahila samitis* (women's organisations) they popularised the notions of maternal and child welfare in respectable Bengali homes. The role of Saroj Nalini Dutt Memorial Association (SNDMA), a prime middle-class Bengali women's organisation founded in 1925, was fundamental in this regard. Dagmar Engels has demonstrated the success of the organisation in gaining access to the district and village homes when compared to similar semi-official efforts made by Vicereine's baby shows or exhibitions.[55] The mouthpiece of the organisation, *Bangalakshmi*, revealed its expanding network in terms of integrating other mahila samitis within its all-encompassing fold and conducting educative lessons on health, hygiene, domestic science, handicrafts, midwifery etc. in the villages and districts of Bengal.

Kalitara Dasgupta, the President of the Madaripur Mahila Samiti, being herself trained in midwifery made personal visits to respectable middle-class homes and imparted education on maternal and infant welfare. Dasgupta also sought the assistance of the local assistant surgeon in arranging classes on maternal and child health that were conducted under the auspices of the Samiti.[56] In the district of Bankura where the rate of infant mortality was stated to be high, special efforts were made to institute a dhai training class where catheters, scissors, nail brushes, carbolic soaps and Vaseline were regularly distributed to the candidates. Baby shows were organised on an annual basis.[57] Similarly, maternal and infant welfare exhibitions were held in Barisal under the auspices of the Barisal Mahila Samiti and with the aid of female doctors and missionaries from local Baptist Mission. These were attended in large numbers by middle-class and lower-middle-class Bengali women across religious divides.[58]

On an all-India level, there were early women's organisations such as *Bharata Mahila Parishad* (Indian Women's Conference) founded in 1904 as part of the National Social Conference and women-only bodies like the *Bharat Stree Mahamandal* (Indian Women's Association, 1910) and the Women's Indian Association (1917). Such associations worked for the advancement of female education, enhancement of social and economic status of widows through primary education and employment, eradication of child marriage and seclusion of women. In the 1920s, the formation of the National Council of Women in India (1925) regarded as the national branch of the International Council of Women and the All-India Women's Conference (AIWC) (1927) constituted important milestones in the formation of a middle-class feminist discourse.[59]

The AIWC, in particular, was instrumental in forging a space for debates and allowed a national network of feminists including eminent medical women to emerge as a powerful pressure group battling for women's issues. From the 1930s, maternity and child welfare work acquired prominence in the agenda of the AIWC, particularly after Dr Muthulakshmi Reddy's presidential address in Lahore in January 1931 where she spelt out the need to solemnly consider the question of providing adequate medical aid to women, allegedly ignored so far by the Central and the local governments. Reddy proposed the creation of a department of health in every Indian province under a senior woman medical officer as the director. The woman medical officer was to start female hospitals in areas where none existed, appoint female medical staff and establish training centres for nurses and midwives. The AIWC, Reddy argued, should also coax the local governments in India into passing legislation akin to the Maternity and Child Welfare Act of 1918 in England in order to safeguard the provision of antenatal and postnatal care of pregnant women and medical aid to women in childbirth. Reddy further stated that it was the responsibility of the members of the AIWC to popularise the work of the maternal and infant welfare centres and ensure that adequate numbers of trained midwives were employed at such centres for assisting women during childbirth.[60]

In 1932, AIWC arranged for the 'training and registration of midwives' on the pattern of similar legislations in England. It emphasised the need for 'propaganda on public health and sanitation'.[61] At its annual session in 1934, the AIWC further passed a resolution urging the need for legislative measures for the compulsory registration of the dhais and the midwives.[62] At its fourteenth session held in Allahabad in 1940, a recommendation was made for the complete elimination of indigenous dhais in the next ten years and their replacement by trained midwives. Also in order to promote professional attendance of every mother at childbirth, provision of maternity beds in rural and urban areas in the 'proportion of one bed for 2,000 of population' was advocated along with the establishment of sufficient numbers of maternity and gynaecological hospitals. The inadequacy of the number of health visitors was mentioned and the need for a 'clear line of demarcation between the duties and responsibilities of the Health Visitor and the trained midwife' was iterated.[63]

The middle-class composition of the AIWC reflected the elitist nature of its demands; Dr Muthulakshmi Reddy's presidential address was a strong proof of such elitism. In prioritising western medical care, Reddy was overly influenced by English examples. Resolutions aimed at marginalising the dhais failed to take cognisance of the fact that the choices of ordinary middle-class women seeking assistance in childbirth were partly dictated by their financial standing and partly by the desire to be attended by a local and familiar dhai who would perform domestic chores at nominal cost. Aparna Basu who was a prominent member of the AIWC and also wrote its history along with Bharati Ray acknowledged the skewed priorities of the organisation and the inability of its members to challenge the basic social, economic and cultural constraints that perpetuated gender subordination in Indian society.[64]

Thus, there were two main levels at which maternal and child welfare schemes were being implemented in colonial Bengal: (a) imperialist efforts at semi-official level and (b) nationalist enterprises at non-official level. Imperial initiatives, despite being indirect, provided the initial motivation; it formed the blueprint on which the foundation of future child welfare schemes was laid and developed in Bengal.

## The local actors

Direct state initiative in women's health and maternal and child welfare work remained peripheral. Financial considerations were central to any changes in the state's policy towards health throughout the nineteenth and the twentieth centuries. Whatever was of little political or economic importance to the empire was brushed aside as insignificant. In the sphere of women's health, for instance, Chapter 2 has shown how financial considerations led the Medical College officials to prioritise training of dhais over that of indigenous male medical students despite the latter's professed interest in learning midwifery and diseases of children as part of medical education. In the early twentieth century, the economic imperatives of the Central Government further prevented any effective measures from being adopted in improving public health in Bengal as in other parts of India. As Ira Klein has argued, 'public health and sanitation were the ugly ducklings of a civil service which rewarded political and military competence, for example, far more highly'.[65] Roger Jeffery while acknowledging that public health and medical services never figured in the high priority list of the colonial state pointed to other factors that might have influenced the medical policy of the government such as the role played by medical bureaucrats, demands of the 'rising political classes' and the 'demands in the market for medical services and education'.[66] Yet the lack of interest of the Central Government was amply evident in its decision to transfer responsibility of public health to the local governments through the Government of India Act, 1919.

Popularly referred to as the 'Montague-Chelmsford reform', the Act of 1919 was a significant milestone in the decentralisation and provincialisation of health administration in India. In the sphere of health, prior to the passage of the act, all power was wielded by the sanitary commissioner and a group of men under him possessing British diplomas of public health. The Act introduced a principle of 'dyarchy' by which certain responsibilities including medical administration and public health were transferred from the Governor-in Council to the popularly elected Indian ministers of local governments who were made responsible to the provincial legislatures. However, the department of finance being in the control of the Centre, the provincial governments were faced with a persistent lack of resources. Also, the lack of coordination between the Central Government and the provincial governments, which was further aggravated by frequent clashes of interests, impeded the smooth working of dyarchy.[67] This defect was corrected only with the establishment of a Central Advisory Board of Health in 1937.[68] On the whole, the Act of 1919 enabled the involvement of Indian ministers in framing and implementing policies in matters relating to medical administration and, in the process, allowed the Central Government to remain indifferent.

Following the decentralisation of public health administration, much of the work pertaining to maternal and infant health in the 1920s came to be conducted at an official level by local bodies, such as municipalities and district boards which now had a greater number of Indian representatives than ever before. Using local self-government files and vernacular sources, the chapter underscores the importance of the 'local' in delivering professional maternity care to Indian women. In Bombay and Madras presidencies, local government and municipalities had taken over the responsibilities of modernising birthing practices much earlier than Bengal. In the case of Madras which was much ahead of the rest of India in western midwifery practices, the local government boards played a significant role from 1875 onwards in providing scholarship and employment to western-trained midwives. By 1917, maternity and child welfare centres were established with women doctors in charge of them.[69] In Bombay presidency, municipal and local government endeavours to improve maternal and infant health commenced in 1901 when free milk was provided to the poor and home-visits were beginning to be made by nurses for instructing mothers on matters pertaining to personal and domestic hygiene. By 1914, at the behest of the Bombay Sanitary Association, three maternity homes with milk depots were established and twelve health visitors were appointed who were to provide antenatal and postnatal care to women and train midwives.[70] In Bengal, the role of the Public Health Department in the sphere of maternal and infant health became visible only in the 1920s whereas that of the Calcutta Municipal Corporation came into view from 1910 onwards. Calcutta evidently followed in the footsteps of Bombay in initiating certain maternal and infant welfare schemes such as establishing maternity homes and appointing health visitors. The maternal and infant welfare schemes of the Corporation, once initiated, struck a chord with the Bengali female population and facilitated the spread of western midwifery in Calcutta.

Interestingly, the Bengal Public Health Report claimed that one of the reasons for the surge in the infant welfare activities in Bengal was the enthusiastic involvement of the District Boards, local bodies and the various municipalities in organising baby shows within the areas under their jurisdiction.[71] In the early 1920s there were five baby clinics in Calcutta and one in Dhaka.[72] Further, it was reported in the annual Bengal public health report of 1925 that twenty-six baby shows were organised in various mufassils towns.[73] It was also optimistically pointed out:

> People are realising the great havoc that ignorance of hygienic rules causes in their homes, and their deep-seated prejudices in matters of infant welfare are being gradually shaken off. People are now more or less willing to spend something on baby clinics and other allied institutions. The work of existing baby clinics continued to be very satisfactory.[74]

By the late 1920s, baby shows were integrated into the schema of health exhibitions and welfare shows that had been organised periodically by municipalities and district boards in Bengal. The nationalist press considered the health exhibitions as 'very good medium of propaganda', the most effective way to remove the 'ignorance of the masses about health matters'.[75]

Despite persistent lack of sufficient funds the mediation of the Indian ministers through local boards and municipalities yielded more sustained results in winning public confidence and in implementing upgraded health measures. The responsibilities taken over by the Calcutta Municipal Corporation from 1909 in working out solutions to curb maternal and infant mortality is a case in point and merits closer attention. It explains how the initiatives of the Corporation triggered a series of initiatives such as establishing domiciliary midwifery services, health visitors and a chain of maternity homes and centres that were designed to improve the quality of professional attendance over childbirth.

The Calcutta Corporation's engagement with health matters had its genesis in the appointment of a permanent health officer in 1886 and more specifically, in the coordination of public health activities under the permanent health officer following the reconstitution of the Corporation in 1899. Eventually, the Calcutta Municipal Act of 1923 widened the sphere of activities of the Corporation. The Corporation claimed to enjoy independent power and responsibilities, with the local government and its health department having no executive power over it.[76] Moreover, the election of an eminent lawyer and nationalist leader like Chittaranjan Das as the mayor of the Corporation in 1924 and a nationalist medical man like Dr Sundari Mohan Das as its Councillor imbued its activities with a distinct nationalist texture. The active involvement of medical men like Dr Haridhan Dutt opened up avenues for experimenting with innovative public health measures.

From 1909, maternal and child health had already began to constitute an area for medical investigation and the launching of welfare schemes. This was a few years before a systematic movement for maternal and child health came into shape in Bengal as elsewhere. The Corporation's contribution to maternal and child health, therefore, constituted a pioneering effort in the first few decades of the twentieth century. In the absence of any Central Government initiatives, it was the only official body showing some degree of social commitment towards maternal and infant health issues.[77]

The maternity and child welfare schemes launched by the Calcutta Municipal Corporation were premised upon coordination between the medical profession and the public health officials that paved the way for the understanding of pregnancy in relation to specific social and economic surroundings in which childbirth took place. In this respect, the role of the Corporation was pivotal to the expansion of the organisational base of midwifery services in Bengal. Under the impact of Corporation initiatives, obstetrics ceased to be grounded solely in hospital training and practices. It moved beyond the confines of medical institutions, into the homes of the pregnant mothers that enabled a more careful monitoring of birth by the medical professionals aided by a professional team of public health workers and western-trained midwives.[78] This coincided with what W. R. Arney terms as the 'monitoring' period in the evolution of the profession of obstetrics. In this phase that began after the Second World War, 'technology changed from a technology of domineering control to a technology of monitoring, surveillance and normalisation'.[79]

The maternity and child welfare scheme of the Corporation chiefly drew the poor and lower-middle-class[80] female population of Bengal within the purview of medical supervision. Schemes such as domiciliary midwifery were evolved with the aim of ensuring improved maternity services and greater accessibility of female patients of all class to western medical care. The consequence was that slums and the lower-middle-class enclaves became the new sites of obstetric research on maternal morbidity. Chapter 2 explained how the foundation of the Dufferin Hospitals was motivated by the need to provide medical assistance to the middle-class purdahnashin women. It implied that the rest of the female population in Bengal lay outside the ambit of medical treatment rendered by the Dufferin hospitals. In this context, the role of the Corporation assumed centrality in drawing the poorer section of the society within the scope of western medical care.

The maternal and infant welfare schemes of the Corporation began with the appointment of two midwives in 1908 that were to look after pregnant women in their houses, free of charge.[81] The next important step was the appointment of female sanitary inspector in 1909. Appointed by the Health Special Committee as an experimental measure on the English model, the duties of the sanitary inspector were varied, ranging from vaccinating young individuals during smallpox epidemic to visiting pregnant women's houses and girls' schools and taking note of the sanitary conditions of schools and the quality of food and milk supply. The General Committee argued in favour of a 'female' sanitary inspector stating:

> It is impossible for any man as an Inspector to gain ready entrance into the interior of homes, see the female members of family, and to get on confidential terms with them regarding their health and that of their children . . . The arguments in favour of such an appointment are tenfold as strong for India as for England.[82]

In 1913 the designation of female sanitary inspector changed to that of 'Health Visitor' in order to make her role more positive and less imposing. According to G. F. McCleary, health visiting 'is a peculiarly

British contribution to the various agencies of the maternal and child welfare movement'.[83] Initially undertaken by English philanthropic women interested in social service, it soon passed into the hands of paid female professional visitors. As McCleary further notes, in the absence of a single qualification which could be deemed as essential for the post of health visitor, most females were employed either as sanitary inspectors with sound knowledge of domestic hygiene and sanitation or as trained nurses or certified midwives. In the case of Calcutta, as the Health Officer of the Corporation observed, the Health Visitor was, in some cases, a qualified medical woman. Her responsibility was specifically outlined as to 'visit and gain the confidence of poor women, and give them simple instructions in elementary hygiene, and to give homely advice as to how to rear their children, etc.'[84]

In the initial years following 1912, imparting scientific training to the dhais constituted an important obligation of the female health visitor of the Corporation. Not only were aseptic scissors and dressings distributed to the dhais, instructions on how to apply ligatures and dressings were also provided. In view of the enormous influence exercised by the dhais on all classes of Bengali female population, the health visitors realised the need to establish 'friendly ties' with them through meetings. The health visitors soon began to contribute towards the restructuring of existing midwifery services in the districts of Bengal. For instance, in December 1915, a female health visitor Miss K. S. Banerjee visited Nityanand Maternity Home in Nabadwip in the Nadia District of Bengal and gave 'practical suggestions' and instructions to its inmates regarding the improvement of the institution. An educated midwife was soon appointed as the Lady Superintendant of the Home.[85]

In 1915, a new class of professionally trained midwives, popularly referred to as the 'corporation midwives', was recruited by the Corporation for domiciliary midwifery services and placed under the supervision of the female health visitor. The preponderant motive was to expunge the 'unprofessional' dhais from the site of birth and reconstitute midwifery into a cohesive professional structure. Despite the initial failure of the corporation midwives to access lower-middle-class homes due to the alleged reluctance of Bengali females to accept the service of 'strange midwives', the scheme slowly began to succeed in limited areas. Within few years the Health Officer confidently noted that 'more than one-fifth of the babies born in Calcutta were delivered by the corporation midwives'.[86]

In 1916, a demand was made by the Health Officer for an increase of staff for midwifery services to four health visitors and sixteen midwives.

A proposal for a 'complete scheme for the whole town' was submitted to the Health Committee in a way that underpinned the emerging coordination between medical profession and the public health officials. Keeping in mind the need to strengthen control over the midwives, provision for free accommodation of the Health Visitor along with the midwives under her supervision was recommended. The proposal was considered by the Health Committee in June 1916 and according to the Health Officer H. M. Crake, 'immediate steps were taken to give effect to their Resolution'. Consequently, midwives and Health Visitors were provided with accommodation within the same premise in order to enforce discipline and better coordination. The number of midwives stood at eight, while the number of Health Visitors was two. A group of four midwives was placed under the supervision of a qualified Health Visitor, each backed by a maternity centre.[87]

The annual reports of the Calcutta Corporation reveal the institutional expansion of the midwifery services into a 'hierarchical' structure with the corporation midwives at the bottom and the medical professionals at the top. In the process, a layered structure of medical control/supervision over the process of birth came to be instituted. It was based not so much on a gendered demarcation of the sphere of action as it was on consolidating grip over the domiciliary midwives by a professionally superior class of medical professionals and Health Visitors (who too were qualified women physicians in certain instances). Thus, the Corporation midwives being part of the professional hierarchy had no independent role. To cite an example, in 1919 under the four Corporation-run maternity centres that came to supervise the delivery cases, it was reported that most patients with 'abnormal' cases were being transferred to the hospital. However, where patients refused to being taken to the hospital, 'local medical men' were called in. Thereupon, a proposal was made before the Health Special Committee to appoint the 'Lady Superintendent' of the Dufferin Hospital as the Consultant Obstetrician with a normal fee for advice and an increased one for operative intervention of any kind. The Committee responded favourably to the decision.[88] An arrangement was eventually made whereby the male obstetricians of the Calcutta Medical Club, a private organisation of the Bengali doctors, agreed to render assistance to the Health Visitors in an event of complication on the payment of a subsidised fee. Thus, a three-layered structure evolved around which the medical profession and public health administration realigned themselves.

The professional structure that was emerging exerted its influence most strongly in instances of pregnancy-related complications when medical/surgical intervention became necessary. For instance, Health Visitor Mrs Clarke's diary reveals how the collaborative efforts of the midwife and the Health Visitor saved maternal lives in cases of abnormalities such as delivery of twins, protracted labour and 'adherent placenta and severe haemorrhage'.[89] Thus, in a certain case of delivery of twins, it was reported that the midwife in course of her official visit to one house discovered that a woman pregnant with twins had delivered one child while the dhai was pulling at the protruding hand of the other. While the corporation midwife was initially prevented by the mother's family from examining the patient who was, by that time, exhausted and wailing, she still managed to inform the Health Visitor of the deteriorating condition of the suffering mother. All the same, the midwife also successfully coaxed the family to allow her to examine the patient. The midwife's timely intervention reportedly brought the Health Visitor to the scene who thereupon performed 'version' and saved the child.[90]

By the 1920s, five maternity centres had been fully established under the auspices of the Calcutta Corporation. Each of them was provided with telephones in order to ensure 'prompt attention to night calls' and ambulance services so that complicated cases could be immediately removed to the hospitals or experts called in on time.[91] Yet much of the maternal and infant welfare work of the Corporation involved extension of medical supervision to the homes of the poor and the lower-middle-class section of the population, the *bustees* (slums) in particular. As the Health Officer pointed out in the annual report, it often entailed conducting delivery in 'insanitary conditions', on the '*kutcha* floor of the *bustee* huts under the most appalling conditions'.[92] In this connection, the need for a well-equipped maternity home for the poor and lower-middle-class Bengali women was earnestly felt. In response to the need, the Buldeodas Maternity Home was established in the northern part of Calcutta in March 1924, more significantly, due to the 'enthusiasm and persistent advocacy' of Dr Haridhan Dutt, the chairman of the Corporation. Dutt's first-hand experience of the maternity and child welfare movement in Bombay and the success of maternity homes in that Presidency caused him to zealously promote the need for similar maternity homes in Calcutta. Hence, the home which was established as a consequence of Dutt's efforts was a three-storeyed building, the first storey being neatly organised into a 'lofty, well-lighted' maternity ward with twenty-two beds, a purdah ward, an admission room and a well-equipped labour room with an adjoining sterilising room.[93] As the Health Officer of the Corporation later recorded, the scheme for the maternity home was started as an experiment, being the first of its kind in Bengal. By 1932, there were four maternity homes in Calcutta, Buldeodas Maternity Home, Chetla Maternity Home, Kidderpore Maternity Home and, lastly, Manicktala Maternity Home.[94]

Within a span of fifteen years, the Buldeodas Maternity Home was extolled by Dr Sundari Mohan Das as the 'best Corporation Maternity Hospital'.[95] A comparison of its annual reports for 1924 and 1934 reveals the growing number of labour cases attended, abnormal labour cases handled and obstetric operations performed, including forceps delivery, version and craniotomy.[96] The first annual report of the Home for the year 1924 revealed the following: the number of 'labour cases' – 353, 'normal labour' – 237, 'abnormal labour' – 116, 'obstetric operations' – 112, forceps delivery – 38, versions – 16 and, lastly, craniotomy – 5 (apart from these, there were a number of minor operations mentioned such as breech, brow and traverse presentations) (see Table 3.1).[97] The 1934 report, on the other hand, showed a steady growth in the number of labour cases admitted. It simultaneously recorded a rise in the number and variety of operative interventions that took place. Thus, the number of 'labour cases' admitted was 2,404, 'normal labour cases' – 1,938, 'abnormal labour cases' – 466, 'Operations' – 270. The report showed a widening of the scope of operative obstetrics by mentioning a variety of surgical measures such as 'forceps', 'evacuation of uterus', 'delivery of normal breech', 'repair of perineum', 'internal version', 'external version', 'episiotomy', 'plugging' and 'replacement of cord' (see Table 3.2).[98]

An overview of the two annual reports of the Corporation provides insight into how the scope and incidence of surgical intervention in childbirth expanded in a span of ten years. In the years following the establishment of the Buldeodas Maternity Home, the ambit of 'practical midwifery' expanded beyond the bounds of the female-run Dufferin hospitals and dispensaries. It managed to lure away patients from the teaching hospitals, a long-standing issue that caused the General Medical Council to withdraw recognition of Indian degrees on grounds of 'defective midwifery training'. Colonel Needham was appointed as an Inspector by the GMC in 1919 with the task of assessing the quality of 'practical' midwifery training imparted by the medical colleges and inspecting the medical examinations conducted by the Indian universities. In his report submitted to the Secretary to the Government of India (Department of Education, Health and Lands) in 1924, the lack of adequate labour cases for practical instructions in midwifery in Calcutta Medical College was partly attributed to the opening of the maternity dispensaries by the Corporation. The

*Table 3.1* A summary of the work done at the Buldeodas Maternity Home, March–December, 1924

| | |
|---|---|
| Patients admitted | 417 |
| Labour cases | 353 |
| Normal labour | 237 |
| Abnormal labour | 116 |
| Obstetrical operations | 112 |
| Forceps | 38 |
| Versions | 16 |
| Placenta praevia | 4 |
| Funis replacement (replacement) | 2 |
| Craniotomy | 5 |
| Removal of placenta and membranes | 15 |
| Plugging for post-partum | 4 |
| Haemorrhage | |
| Ante-partum haemorrhage | 1 |
| Breech | 12 |
| Transverse presentations | 12 |
| Brow presentation (which was converted into face and delivered) | 1 |
| Emptying of the uterus of foetus or products of conception in abortion and miscarriages) | 15 |
| Twins | 10 |
| Of the 363 babies born in the maternity home | |
| Born alive and discharged well on the tenth day | 291 |
| Weakly babies born alive but dying within ten days | 7 |
| Premature non-viable babies born alive (heart acting) | 10 |
| Dead and macerated babies | 40 |
| Infant patients | 11 |
| Fractured membranes | 1 |
| Septic cords | 1 |
| Convulsion and green diarrhoea | 1 |
| Parietal abscess | 1 |
| Diarrhoea and debility | 3 |
| Torn cord | 1 |
| Maternal mortality | 2 |
| Toxaemia of pregnancy (eclampsia) | 1 |
| Heart disease | 1 |

Source: Report of the Health Officer of Calcutta, 1924

Corporation responded by passing a resolution that allowed students to attend, labour cases in their dispensaries, provided they were summoned by the resident obstetrician and the patient gave permission.[99] In 1939 the growing popularity of the maternity homes was attributed to the 'increase of hospital-mindedness of the public', so that 'there is greater and greater demand for admission of emergent labour cases and the beds are filled up to the utmost capacity of the wards, leaving

*Table 3.2* A summary of the work done at the Buldeodas Maternity Home, March–December, 1934

| | | | |
|---|---|---|---|
| **New admissions** | 2,748 | Anaemia of pregnancy | 24 |
| a) Labour cases | 2,523 | | |
| b) Other cases | 225 | | |
| **Full-term labour cases** | 2,404 | Pregnancy with fever | 28 |
| a) Normal | 1,938 | | |
| b) Abnormal | 466 | | |
| Abortions and premature labour | 119 | Pregnancy with pneumonia | 3 |
| Operations | 270 | Pregnancy with other complication | 10 |
| Maternal mortality | 11 | Anti-partum haemorrhage | 8 |
| Infant mortality including stillbirths and macerated foetus | 236 | Post-partum haemorrhage | 8 |
| **Types of operation** | | Placenta praevia | 7 |
| Forceps | 24 | Transverse presentation | 15 |
| Manual removal of placenta | 16 | Face presentation | 12 |
| Craniotomy | 9 | Artificial rupture of membranes | 5 |
| Evacuation of foetus | 41 | **Causes of maternal mortality** | |
| Delivery of abnormal breech | 16 | Pneumonia | 1 |
| Repair of perineum | 102 | Eclampsia | 3 |
| Internal version | 10 | Admitted in moribund condition | 1 |
| Plugging | 10 | Septicaemia | 1 |
| Intrauterine wash | 9 | Post-partum haemorrhage | 1 |
| Episiotomy | 6 | Anaemia of pregnancy | 3 |
| **Abnormal cases** | | **Infant mortality** | |
| Forceps delivery | 24 | Premature | 46 |
| Delayed labour | 33 | Macerated | 105 |
| Albuminuria | 42 | Convulsions | 4 |
| Eclampsia | 24 | Congenital heart | 2 |
| Breech | 55 | Congenital defect | 1 |
| Twins | 27 | Diarrhoea | 2 |

Source: Report of the Health Officer of Calcutta, 1934

no space for the admission of prospective mothers'. The Buldeodas Maternity Home, in particular, was compared to a 'pilgrim shed rather than a hospital, fulfilling modern ideas of civilisation and sanitation'.[100]

In 1926, the Corporation assumed the responsibility of training the nurses for midwifery services and other subjects. Accordingly, a Nurses' Training Class was instituted. The pupils were selected by the Health Officer on the basis of a preliminary examination in general knowledge. After selection they were instructed by four lecturers appointed by the Public Health Committee. The training class on gaining popularity was eventually affiliated to the Bengal Nursing Council which was brought into being by the government in 1934 for the recognition of qualified nurses.[101]

While the burgeoning influence of the Corporation in implementing public health measures pointed towards decentralisation of health administration in India with increasing power being now wielded by the Indians, the foundation of the All India Institute of Hygiene and Public Health (AIIHPH) in 1934 indicated a parallel trend of internationalisation of health. Yet at the same time, empowering Indians in matters pertaining to public health administration remained at the heart of the initiative to form the AIIHPH. David Arnold has effectively charted the chequered history of the maternity and child welfare section of the Institute. According to Arnold, lack of colonial state interest and the persistent shortage of finances hindered the effective organisation and staffing of that particular section.[102] Nevertheless, the maternity and child welfare section represented an important step towards training Indian men and, especially, women in reproductive health.[103] It was part of the broader scheme evolved by the provincial governments for training the Indians in public health and providing them with higher diplomas. Such arrangements were made in order to enable the Indians trained in their own countries to become 'Health Officers of the first class'.[104]

The need for providing 'specialised' training to Indians as public health workers was stressed in 1925 by J. D. Graham, the Public Health Commissioner with the Government of India in the following words: 'This is a work which has to be done for the benefit of the Indians . . . to be effective it must carry conviction and establish its position against immemorial conservatism and tradition; it must therefore be done by Indians.' Not only was the involvement of Indians stressed, but the specific need for a 'careful system of specialised training in institutes or schools devoted to public health teaching and research' was reiterated.[105] Graham's views were shared by John Megaw, the head of the Calcutta School of Tropical Medicine and Hygiene. It soon came to be appreciated by W. S. Carter, Associate Director of the Rockefeller Foundation.

The intervention of the Rockefeller Foundation in the foundation of the AIIHPH is a classic example of internationalisation of public health in India even as efforts were made to ensure greater involvement of Indians in health administration at the local and provincial levels. The international Health Division of the Rockefeller Foundation, as it turned out, assisted in the initial foundation of the AIIHPH in 1934 although the Foundation was soon fated to fall out with the Indian Research Fund Association over issues of management and administration of the newly founded institute that severely jeopardised its functioning. After 1945, the institute was left to fend for itself.[106] Previously, the Rockefeller Foundation had successfully established a chair at the School of Tropical Medicine, Calcutta, in 1916.

In the case of AIIHPH however, the success of the Rockefeller Foundation was rather muddled. At the initial stage, Carter's empathetic intervention and subsequent meetings with the Government of India enabled the setting up of the institute in the extremely troubled times in which it was founded. In the wake of the Great Depression of 1929, it was agreed that the Rockefeller Foundation would provide for the building and initial set up of the institute while the Government of India would pay for its recurring cost of staff and maintenance of the building. 'Maternity and Child Welfare and School Hygiene' constituted one of the six sections that were opened along with other sections such as 'Public Health Administration', 'Sanitary Engineering' and 'Biochemistry and Nutrition'. It remained one of the sections with a turbulent history of initial neglect and sustained underfunding. The inability of the government to meet the expenses led Graham to eventually stop the funding of the maternity and child welfare section. Consequently, the financial responsibility of the section was taken over by voluntary bodies like Dufferin Fund and the Red Cross Association of India and much later by the Calcutta Municipal Corporation, Calcutta Health Week Committee, the Calcutta Footballers' Association and the Turf Club.[107]

The women doctors of the WMS who were attached to the AIIHPH took responsibility of training students for diploma in maternity and child welfare course (DMCW) started in 1933 by the Calcutta School of Tropical Medicine and Hygiene. One of the medical women of the senior cadre of the service, Dr Jean M. Orkney, was appointed as the Professor of Maternity and Child Welfare in 1934.[108] In the first year, seventy lectures were recorded to have been delivered on various aspects of maternity and child welfare work, school medical services, infant and child development, child psychology etc. In addition, 180 hours were allotted to field work, administrative experience and other upgraded tasks such as clinical work and research writing. However, within two years, Orkney as the Head of the section lamented the lack of students for the course which led to the course being stalled for a few years. Despite such setbacks, there were a few notable accomplishments of the AIIHPH. The first was the opening of a maternity and child welfare centre in 1935 in ward 8 (north-central part) of Calcutta where the steady increase in clinic attendance was largely due to a strong network of antenatal, postnatal and intra-natal services. Instituting mother-craft lessons and nursery school formed part of the centre's duties. The second achievement was the introduction of maternity and child welfare scheme in the Clive Jute Mill, also in 1935. It was launched with a view to undertake investigative enquiry into the health and nutrition of women jute mill workers under the industrial conditions and the impact of such conditions on the reproductive functions of the mother and the health of the infant in the first year of birth.[109] It was appreciated in the nationalist press as a 'move in the right direction'.[110]

Outside the framework of the AIIHPH and its manifold activities, the Rockefeller Foundation committed itself to initiating a rural health unit in Bengal as it had been doing in Ceylon, Burma and other Indian provinces, although maternal and child welfare activities were not the central concerns of such endeavours. In Bengal, the Rockefeller Foundation financed the setting up of a rural health training centre at Singur in 1939 which was conceived as a focal training centre for health visitors and sanitary inspectors. The Singur Health Unit represented a collaborative venture between the Government of Bengal and the Foundation and although affiliated to AIIHPH, the latter made no financial contribution whatsoever. The Singur Health Unit eventually came to be known as SN Mallick Maternity Home and Model Health Unit, after the widow of an eminent government official made generous donation of land and money for the construction and maintenance of the health centre. However, the actual functioning of the Health Unit was severely hampered by the daily bickering between local authorities and the Rockefeller Foundation over minor administrative and financial issues.[111]

The question that remains central to the discussion on maternal and infant mortality schemes introduced by the Public Health Department and Calcutta Corporation is: Was there any noticeable reduction in the infant and maternal mortality rates in the period between 1910s and 1947? The Calcutta Corporation reports revealed that in the period between 1900 and 1935, infant mortality rate fell from 443 per 1,000 to 239 per 1,000. Except for the years 1943–44 and 1944–45, infant mortality rate showed a downward trend. Yet, as the health officer of the Corporation continued to point out, defective registration of births and deaths often accounted for inaccuracies in the calculation of mortality figures.[112] However, infant mortality rates in the rural areas, as shown by the public commissioners' reports in the

1930s and 1940s, continued to be high with occasional decline in certain years.[113] Maternal mortality rates, on the other hand, were published from the 1930s in particular. The Public Health Commissioners noted in 1938 that female death rates for the ages between fifteen and forty years were higher than male death rates, which were recognised to be chiefly due to childbearing causes.[114] The infant mortality rate was higher amongst the Muslims than the Hindus in the entire period under review. The Health Officer of the Calcutta Corporation stated in his reports that the observance of purdah was stricter amongst the Muslims than amongst the Hindus which often led to a rejection of medical advice and care offered by western-trained health visitors and midwives.[115] This compels one to assume (in the absence of sufficient evidences) that despite the Muslim reformers' attempts to popularise western medical practice amongst the Muslim women, the majority of lower-class Muslim women remained entrenched in decadent practices of purdah and, hence, were perhaps more resistant to western medicine than the middle-class educated Muslim females and the Hindu bhadramahila at large.

## The growing 'Hospital Habit' in the interwar years

In a statistical survey on maternal mortality conducted in 1934 by Dr Kedarnath Das under the auspices of the Indian Statistical Institute in the Eden Hospital which was based on records of maternal deaths for the years 1850–1901 and 1902–15, an increase in the attendance by 'Bengali Hindu' females was noted. The increased trend of hospitalisation was partly attributed to the rise in population and partly to transformations in the habits of the people, the growing recognition of the importance of hospitals and, lastly, the gradual fading away of the prejudices preventing Hindu females from being sent to the hospital for childbirth. Not only complicated delivery, but normal cases were also recorded to have been brought to the hospital. It was further observed that maternal mortality was lower when normal cases were admitted to the hospital. This fuelled the expectation that the gradual increase in the number of normal cases being brought to the hospital could lead to a 'steady fall' in maternal death rates.[116] This was in startling contrast to the claims made at the turn of the century about the bulk of the Bengali population, with the exception of those who were 'very poor', being averse to seeking treatment at the public hospitals.[117] Considering the fact that such claims were based on Bengal Administration Reports of the years 1897–99, Das's findings might appear to be an expression of robust optimism with little bearing on reality. Yet certain trends which became visible in the interwar years and thereafter seemed to vindicate Das's claim.

The soaring popularity of the Buldeodas Maternity Home in the 1920s is a case in point. It demonstrates the extent to which the western medical discourse was internalised by the middle class, nationalist politicians and medical men and was disseminated to the relatively poorer sections of the Bengali society. As the higher incidence of surgical intervention in the maternity home reveals, the shift in the site of birth from home to hospital gradually 'normalised' operative intervention under proper medical supervision. Within two years of the foundation of the Buldeodas Maternity Home, Chittaranjan Seva Sadan, another hospital for the lower-class women and children, was established on similar principles, albeit outside the jurisdiction of the Corporation. The objective behind the foundation of Seva Sadan was to celebrate the legacy of Chittaranjan Das, the mayor of the Corporation, following his death in 1925. Guided by the ideology of providing 'relief to the poor and suffering womanhood and of imparting instructions to women' Das had created a Trust of the whole of his property prior to his death. Following his death, the mediation of Mahatma Gandhi helped raise a hefty sum of eight lakh rupees which was utilised to build a women's hospital for the poor and the lower middle class in Calcutta. The history of the hospital from 1927 to 1941 was marked by expansion of the building to start an outpatient department for treatment of women and children and more notably to accommodate more patients. In 1936, a separate paediatric ward was erected under the name of 'Chittaranjan Sishu Sadan'.[118] *Bangalakshmi*, the prominent women's journal, noted with pride how each female patient was treated with tenderness and care. The diet and treatment of each patient was reported to have been meticulously taken care of by 'two lady doctors and one experienced Indian matron'.[119]

There was a perceptible shift in the ideology guiding the foundation of the latter day maternity homes. Unlike the foundation of the Dufferin chain of hospitals in the 1880s, propelled by the need to absorb purdahnashin women into the colonial medical discourse, the maternity homes established in the wake of the maternity and infant welfare movement in Bengal sought to accommodate women of 'all classes' within the scope of medical science as a form of service to the nation. Neal Edward, while conducting research on maternal mortality in Calcutta for the year 1936, referred to the 'growing popularity of institutional delivery' in the city.[120] Apart from the Eden Hospital and the Dufferin Hospitals, other institutions such as the Campbell Medical School, National Medical School and Calcutta Medical School came to accommodate pregnant women from the middle and lower classes for both obstetric (normal/abnormal labour) cases and gynaecological complications. In 1936, a charitable hospital for women attached to the Ramakrishna Medical College for Women was inaugurated by the prominent women of Calcutta with a view 'that their students might acquire experience in the treatment of patients and their diagnosis'. The hospital was reported to be in demand even before it was formally inaugurated.[121] In a similar tone, the principal of the Carmichael Medical College complained about the 'great rush for admission into the Maternity Wards of the Hospital in spite of the increase in the number of beds lately . . . It is becoming increasingly difficult to provide for this daily extra accommodation'.[122]

Finally, a speech delivered by the Governor of Bengal during the opening of a maternity ward at the Howrah General Hospital in September 1937 succinctly captures the ideology guiding the trend towards hospitalisation of childbirth. The Governor remarked:

> The inauguration of this Maternity Ward to-day has a far wider significance than the opening of a new block of nineteen beds. It marks your recognition of a profound and growing change in outlook on the part not only of women but of men also, for men also have their part to play in seeing that their wives and daughters at this most crucial moment of human life have the benefit of the best that medical science can give. Those who have contributed to this project whether by money or by service have kindled yet another torch to light the path for the rising generation.[123]

## Critiquing the maternal and infant welfare schemes

Existing historical works have amply indicated how the colonial state's initiatives in matters of women's reproductive health were largely politically motivated and, hence, confined to the working classes in certain organised sectors such as the mines, jute mills and tea plantations. Even in those specific sectors the steps taken in the form of starting a chain of maternity and child welfare centres in the various mills or prohibition of female underground labour in 1929 were far from adequate. Throughout the 1920s and 1930s, the government was wary of expanding social and health services by instituting maternity leave or paying cash compensation to the working-class mothers. Instead it brought the childbearing practices of such mothers within public scrutiny.[124] Perhaps the only substantial government intervention came in 1939 with the passing of the Bengal Maternity Benefit Act designed chiefly for the female workers in factories and jute mills. The Act was implemented with the objective of 'regulating the employment of women in factories' during certain period before and after childbearing and to provide maternity benefits to them. The government further elaborated the 'Maternity Benefit Scheme' in an official report. It defined the nature of services the female labourers were to have access to such as maternity and child health welfare centres under competent health officers and doctors, baby clinics, mother craft classes, availability of hospitals in tea gardens, supply of milk and food, a certain amount of bonus to the mother during birth etc. Similarly, in the rural areas the government was reported in 1940 to have planned to start maternity and child welfare clinics in each of the 600 *thanas* (police station areas) that existed in the whole of Bengal. However, for such a scheme to take shape, the rural people were to bear half the expenses. As a beginning, the government took upon itself the task of training the health visitors and raising the standards of dhais whose dominance in midwifery could not be entirely done away with.[125]

Piecemeal efforts to regulate the training and activities of the midwives and provide for their compulsory registration were made in 1934 through the Bengal Nurses and Midwives Registration Act.[126] The Act officially came into force in February 1936. But the inadequacy of the Act in producing sufficient number of registered midwives remained a focal point of criticism in the following years.[127] Need for adequate government funding to promote effective dhai training continued to be voiced during the budget discussions in Bengal Legislative Council in the 1940s.[128] In 1941 Dr Sundari Mohan Das advised the government to train the traditional dhais instead of getting rid of them altogether so that 'while these women will not be absolutely stranded, the situation created by the paucity of trained midwives will be somewhat eased'. Also it was believed that 'given a course of training these indigenous dais were likely to turn out quite efficient as the profession, in their case being mostly hereditary, they got something like a natural aptitude for the work, which combined with the training was to give very good results'.[129] The key idea was therefore to co-opt the dhais into the modern maternal health care system by curbing their autonomy and reducing them to mere appendages.[130]

Condemning government's apathy, concerned medical men argued, 'The duties and responsibilities of guardianship of the Nation's children must be shared by individuals and by the State.'[131] All this led to the appointment of a special committee by the Central Advisory Board of Health in 1937. The committee was assigned the task of drawing up a report on the maternity and child welfare work in India. The report was subsequently published leading to fifty-three recommendations being made on administration, coordination and supervision of maternity and child welfare services including the training of staff.[132]

Following the Report of 1938, a new committee known as the Health Survey and Development Committee popularly referred to as the Bhore Committee was appointed by the Government of India on 18 October 1943 under the chairmanship of Sir Joseph Bhore. It consisted of twenty-five distinguished Indian personalities including obstetricians Dr Hilda Lazarus of the WMS and Dr L. S. Mudaliar. Its chief task was to conduct a broad survey of the health conditions in British India and make recommendations for future. It was to be the basis of a 'National Health Plan'. The findings of the Bhore Committee in 1946 confirmed the inadequacy of the existing maternity services in the country as a whole. For instance, the committee found out that the number of practising midwives in the whole of British India was 5,000, whereas the actual requirement was that of 100,000 midwives for conducting approximately ten million births in the country on the basis of 'one midwife to 100 births'. In view of the enormity of the task of quickly training a large number of midwives in a short span of time, an 'interim measure' of training the dhais and permitting them to conduct deliveries under 'proper supervision' was proposed. Even the number of health visitors was considered 'inadequate' and the number of women doctors equally insufficient.[133]

The committee recommended the raising of the age of marriage for girls, improving the standard of living and, lastly, regulating fertility through self-control. Most of its recommendations were met with protest from the members, while some were not implemented due to the financial incapacity of the government, a problem which persisted in the post-colonial period. However, as David Arnold has argued, it constituted a more decisive proof of the fact that 'maternal and infant health had begun to move from margins of public health concerns into the mainstream'.[134]

The indifference of the state to the increasing infant mortality in districts and rural areas was thoroughly condemned in the press in the 1940s. Allegations that the maternity and child welfare scheme had merely touched the 'fringe' of the problem continued to be made by nationalist politicians and medical professionals. Mira Datta Gupta, a well-known social activist on women's issues and also a member of the Legislative Assembly, ruefully pointed out that the 'blackest spots' in Bengal were the rural areas where 'poor mothers' 'were dying in increasing number unattended and uncared for'. Government's indifference, in her opinion, was the chief cause behind the escalating rates of maternal and infant mortality and hence had to be condemned by all. As late as 1945 the government was reminded in course of the Bengal Legislative Council debates, of its non-committal approach towards maternal and child welfare work that led to most of the maternity centres and homes being founded at the behest of the local self-governing institutions.[135]

Lack of government initiative led to existing hospitals and maternity wards being left in a state of neglect even when they were highly in demand. Neal Edward's research on the causes of maternal mortality in Calcutta in the 1930s revealed that 'there is no question that the present *demand* exceeds the supply and as a higher standard of maternal care develops, this demand will undoubtedly increase, for the *need* very far exceeds the supply' (emphasis original). Edward went on to recommend that:

> The limitations, defects and even danger of small inefficient institutions, whether hospitals or maternity homes, must also be recognised. When such institutions are overcrowded or staffed inadequately, or are without proper arrangements for segregation of septic cases, they may be a source of danger, especially to women in a poor state of health with lowered resistance to infection. Regulations for the supervision and control of such institutions admitting maternity cases are therefore required.[136]

## Conclusion

To sum up, the chapter has analysed how midwifery services in Bengal were expanded and reorganised around maternity and child welfare schemes in the interwar years. It has shown the significance of the nationalist rhetoric of motherhood in the writings of Bengali medical men on maternal and infant welfare. Also concerns for racial degeneration played a pivotal role in opening up new and more patriotic ways of reconceptualising the importance of maternal and infant health in the growth of nation, although the solution was sought in medical terms, by expanding the limits of professionalised obstetrics. It led to professional supervision and institutional delivery being perceived as less hazardous ways of giving birth and preventing unnecessary wastage of infant and maternal life.

The chapter has highlighted the key players in the domain of maternal and infant health in Bengal: the Calcutta Corporation and the district municipalities, voluntary bodies like the Red Cross Society, professional bodies like the Bengal Obstetric and Gynaecological Society and newly established public health training institutions like the AIIHPH, all of which were outside the orbit of direct government control. In the process, the chapter has brought out the fragmented and apathetic nature of government initiative in promoting maternity and child welfare programmes.

Despite lack of state support causing much of the maternity welfare work being undertaken by the voluntary bodies and municipalities, the fact remains that by the 1940s, midwifery and modern maternity services had expanded in the city of Calcutta and adjoining districts. They had broadened enough to accommodate more patients from all classes into a burgeoning number of maternity homes and hospitals under the supervision of health professionals. And more importantly such medical services were extended to the slums and lower-middle-class enclaves in Calcutta. Thus, the popularity of institutional delivery in Bengal can be clearly traced to this period.

While inaugurating a maternity and child welfare exhibition by the Calcutta Corporation in 1941, an eminent medical man from Bombay, Mangaldas V. Mehta, remarked that opening maternity homes for the medical assistance of pregnant women or training the indigenous dhai constituted the initial step in the Maternity and Child Welfare Movement. The more comprehensive programme would entail eradication of prejudices and ignorance amongst the masses through proper education. Mehta, therefore, proposed to focus on the 'preventive' side of obstetrics as the more advanced step in maternity and child welfare work. This, according to him, was 'prenatal' care which formed the essence of the preventive side of obstetrics and the most potent instrument to combat maternal and infant mortality.[137] The next chapter will, therefore, analyse how the doctrine of antenatal care was appropriated by the medical profession in Bengal to redefine the nature of its control over the birthing process.

## Notes

1 Quoted in P.G. Thomas, 'The National Health and Baby Week: Its Importance and the Reasons Why We Should Help It', *The Calcutta Municipal Gazette*, May 1927, 57.
2 'Maternity and Child Welfare in India', *Calcutta Medical Journal*, Vol.32, No.8, August 1937, 392.
3 'Medical Profession and Maternal and Child Welfare', *Calcutta Medical Journal*, Vol.41, No.6, June 1944, 198.
4 Anna Davin, 'Imperialism and Motherhood', *History Workshop*, No.5, Spring 1978, 9–65.
5 G.F. McCleary, *The Maternity and Child Welfare Movement*, London: P.S. King & Son, 1935, 15–16.
6 The Swadeshi movement was an offshoot of the anti-partition movement that crystallised around the Viceroy's decision to partition Bengal citing administrative reasons. The Swadeshi movement started with an economic motive to promote and stimulate the growth of indigenous industries in Bengal, but went on to become the economic, political and spiritual weapon of the Bengalis symbolising the desire for independence. The years following the Swadeshi movement were marked by strong

nationalist ideas amongst the Bengalis. For details see Sumit Sarkar, *The Swadeshi Movement in Bengal, 1903–1908*, New Delhi: Permanent Black, 2010; S.N. Sen, *History of Freedom Movement in India, 1857–1947*, New Delhi: New Age Internationals Publishers 1997.

7  For instance, see Donald Paterson, 'Maternity and Child Welfare Services in Their Relation to Public Health', *British Medical Journal*, Vol.1, No.3773, April 1933, 742–744.
8  *Bengal Public Health Report, 1925*, Calcutta: Bengal Secretariat Book Depot, 65.
9  Jane Lewis, *The Politics of Motherhood: Child and Maternal Welfare in England, 1900–1939*, London: Croom Helm, 1980, Introduction.
10 Bamandas Mukherjee 'Second All India Obstetric and Gynaecological Congress Bombay', *Medical Digest*, Vol.6, No.4, January 1938, 142.
11 Ibid.
12 'Indigenous Health Science', *Cikitsa Sammilani*, May–June, 1885 as translated in Pradip Kumar Bose, *Health and Society in Bengal: A Selection from Late 19th-Century Bengali Periodicals*, New Delhi: Sage, 2006.
13 Tanika Sarkar, 'Nationalist Iconography: Image of Women in 19th Century Bengali Literature', *Economic and Political Weekly*, Vol.22, No.47, 1987, 2011–2015.
14 Jasodhara Bagchi, 'Representing Nationalism: Ideology of Motherhood in Colonial Bengal', *Economic and Political Weekly*, Vol.25, Nos.42–43, 1990, 66. Indira Chowdhury has also argued that, 'The bhadralok invention of the goddess of the motherland or the Bharat Mata combined different attributes of both Durga and Kali'. See Indira Chowdhury, *The Frail Hero and Virile History: Gender and the Politics of Culture in Colonial Bengal*, Delhi: Oxford University Press, 1998, Chapter 4.
15 Margaret M. Urquhart, *Women of Bengal: A Study of the Hindu Pardanashins of Calcutta*, Second Edition, Calcutta: Association Press YMCA, 1926, 83–84.
16 Bharati Ray, 'Women of Bengal: Transformation in Ideas and Ideals, 1900–1947', *Social Scientist*, Vol.19, No.5/6, 1991, 19.
17 Manisha Roy, *Bengali Women*, Chicago and London: Chicago University Press, 1975, 166–167.
18 'Adarsha Janani (Ideal Mother)', *Bamabodhini Patrika*, Vol.8, No.101, December 1871, 261–264, see 262.
19 'Ma (Mother)', *Bamabodhini Patrika*, No.256, February 1887, 290–293. Another series of essays making similar points which began to be published in *Bamabodhini* from September was 'Matribhakti o Matriupasana e Santaner Mukti (Son's Liberation Lies in Devotion to Mother)', *Bamabodhini Patrika*, No.356, September 1894, 132–134.
20 Sarkar, *The Swadeshi Movement*, 419–420.
21 See Debendranath Mukherji, *Khokar Ma* (The Baby's Mother: Hints to a Mother on the Feeding, Rearing and Diseases of Infants), Calcutta: Aryan Press, 1902; Sarachchandra Dhar, *Adarsha Janani*, Dhaka: Nagendrachandra Roy, 1914; Jogendra Lal Chowdhury, *Adarsha Janani* (Ideal Mother), Calcutta: Swarna Press, 1927; Anurupa Devi, *Sisumangal* (Instruction in Child Welfare and Rearing of Children), Calcutta: Bodhodoy Press, 1926. Apart from individual pamphlets, series of articles on infant rearing

were published, for instance, see '*Santan Palan* (Child Rearing)', *Svasthya Samacara*, Vol.4, No.2, June 1915; Vol.4, No.3, July 1915; Vol.3, No.6, September 1915; Vol.4, No.8, November 1915; Also see '*Sisupalan* (Child Rearing)', *Svasthya Samacara*, Vol.5, No.3, July 1916, 76–79; '*Jananir Prati* (An Address to the Mother), *Svasthya Samacara*', Vol.8, No.7, October 1919, 148–150; Vol.4, No.3, July 1915; Vol.3, No.6, September 1915; Vol.4, No.8, November 1915.

22 Davin, 'Imperialism and Motherhood'.

23 Ramesh Chandra Ray, 'Child Welfare', *Indian Medical Record*, Vol.39, September 1919.

24 In the later years, A.C. Chatterjee, the Director of Public Health singled out the role of bhadramahila in promoting national health and welfare by imagining her in multiple roles of mother, wife, 'head of the family', 'doctor of medicine', 'public health nurse', 'sick nurse', midwife, social worker and teacher of health education. A.C. Chatterjee, 'Women's Role in National Health', *Calcutta Municipal Gazette*, June 1941, 211.

25 Ray, 'Child Welfare'.

26 Samita Sen, *Women and Labor in Late Colonial India: The Bengal Jute Industry*, Cambridge: Cambridge University Press, 1999, 149.

27 Dagmar Engels, 'The Politics of Childbirth: British and Bengali Women in Contest, 1890–1930', in *Beyond Purdah? Women in Bengal, 1890–1930*, New Delhi: Oxford University Press, 1996, 123–161.

28 L.S.S. O'Malley, *Census of India (Vol.VI): City of Calcutta, Part I*, Calcutta: Bengal Secretariat Book Depot, 1913, 2.

29 H.M. Crake, *Report of the Health Officer of Calcutta*, Calcutta: The Corporation Press, 1914, 5.

30 'Bengal Legislative Council Interpretations: Mortality of Infants Under One Year in Bengal', *The Amrita Bazar Patrika*, 1 April 1919.

31 Engels, 'Politics of Childbirth'.

32 '*Sisu Marak* (Infant Mortality)', *Svasthya Samacara*, Vol.8, No.3, July 1920, 53.

33 Editorial, *The Amrita Bazar Patrika*, 25 April 1914.

34 Sarah Hodges, 'Indian Eugenics in an Age of Reform', in Sarah Hodges, ed. *Reproductive Health in India: History, Politics, Controversies*, Delhi: Orient Longman, 2006.

35 'National Health – How Marriage Affects It', *Svasthya*, January–February 1901, as translated by Pradip Kumar Bose, *Health and Society in Bengal: A Selection from Late 19th-Century Bengali Periodicals*, New Delhi: Sage, 2006, 134–135.

36 U.N. Mukherji, *Hindus: A Dying Race*, Calcutta: M. Bannerjee, 1909.

37 Pradip Kumar Dutta, *Carving Blocs: Communal Ideology in Early Twentieth-Century Bengal*, New Delhi: Oxford University Press, 1999, Chapter 1.

38 Such articles portraying infant mortality as reflection of the deterioration of race appeared *in Svasthya Samacara* and also in women's magazines such as *Bharati*. For instance see '*Jatikkhoy o Sisu mrityu* (Racial Deterioration and Infant Mortality)', *Bharati*, Vol.43, No.10, January 1919.

39 '*Bibahopon o Svasthya* (Dowry and Health)', *Svasthya*, Vol.5, Nos.6 and 7, September–October, 1901.

40 K.C. Chaudhuri, 'The Problem of Infant Welfare in Calcutta', *Calcutta Municipal Gazette*, Fourth Health Number, March 1932, 62.

41 Ramesh Chandra Ray, 'Child Welfare: Anti-Venereal Campaign', *Indian Medical Record*, Vol.39, September 1919, 161.

42 For instance, one Dr Panchanan Basu in an essay entitled '*Sisumrityur Protikar* (Ways to Arrest Infant Mortality) explained how diseases like malaria or tuberculosis which afflicted the mother during pregnancy resulted in the birth of weak and diminutive children. See Dr Panchanan Basu, '*Sisumrityur Protikar* (Ways to Arrest Infant Mortality)', *Svasthya Samacara*, Vol.15, No.4, July 1926. See for instance, '*Sisu Marak* (Infant Mortality)', Vol.8, No.3, July 1919; '*Bange Sisu Mrityur Karon* (Infant Mortality in Bengal and Its Reasons)', *Svasthya Samacara*, Vol.8, No.6, September 1919; '*Sisu-mrityu o tahar karon* (Infant Mortality and Its Reasons)', *Svasthya Samacara*, Vol.8, No.11, February 1919.

43 Mrinalini Sinha, ed. *Mother India: Selections from the Controversial 1927 Text*, Delhi: Kali for Women Press, 1998, 3.

44 Quoted in Laxmibai Rajwade, 'The Indian Mother and Her Problems', in *Our Cause: A Symposium by Indian Women*, Allahabad: Kitabistan, 1938, 80.

45 '*Sisur Pranraksha* (Saving the Life of Infant)', *Svasthya*, Vol.4, No.10, 1916, 307–310. The article was originally published in another Bengali periodical *Prabasi*.

46 Thomas, 'The National Health and Baby Week'.

47 NAI, Foreign and Political Department, General Branch, September 1920, Part B.

48 Ibid.

49 Margaret Balfour and Ruth Young, *The Work of Medical Women*, Oxford: Oxford University Press, 1929, 150.

50 Balfour and Young, *The Work of Medical Women*, 145.

51 Ibid.

52 Thomas, 'The National Health and Baby Week', 58.

53 For more on baby shows see Sujata Mukherjee, 'Disciplining the Body? Health Care for Women and Children in Early Twentieth Century Bengal', in Deepak Kumar, ed. *Disease and Medicine in India: A Historical Overview*, New Delhi: Tulika, 2001.

54 Kaliprasanna Ray, '*Matrimangal o Sisumangal Saptaha* (Maternal Welfare and Baby Welfare Week)', *Svasthya Samacara*, Vol.14, No.10, January 1926, 315–316.

55 Engels, 'Politics of Childbirth'.

56 '*Mahila Samiti Sangbad: Madaripur* (News from Women's Organization: Madaripur)', *Bangalakshmi*, B.S. 1334–35(1927–28), 142–143.

57 'Bankura', *Bangalakshmi*, B.S. 1334–35 (1927–28), 143.

58 'Barisal', *Bangalakshmi*, B.S. 1334–35 (1927–28), 144–145.

59 Radha Kumar, *The History of Doing: An Illustrated Account of Movements for Women's Rights and Feminism in India, 1800–1900*, New Delhi: Zubaan, 1993, Chapter 4.

60 S. Muthulakshmi Reddy, 'Presidential Address', *All India Women's Conference*, Fifth Session, Lahore, January, 1931, 34–35.

61 Memorandum", *AIWC*, 7th Annual Report, Lucknow, 1933, 140.

62 Annual Report, *AIWC*, Ninth Session, Karachi, January, 1935, 121.

63 Annual Report, *AIWC*, Fourteenth Session, Allahabad, January 1940, 61–62.

64 Aparna Basu and Bharati Ray, ed. *Women's Struggle: A History of the All India Women's Conference, 1927–1990*, Delhi: Manohar, 1990, 143.

65 Ira Klein, 'Death in India, 1871–1921', *The Journal of Asian Studies*, Vol.32, No.4, August 1973, 656.

66 Roger Jeffery, *The Politics of Health in India*, Berkeley and Los Angeles, London: University of California Press, 1988, 102.

67 N. Jayapalan, *Modern Governments and Constitutions*, Vol.II, New Delhi: Atlantic Publishers, 2002.

68 Kabita Ray, *History of Public Health: Colonial Bengal, 1921–1947*, Calcutta: K.P. Bagchi, 1998.

69 David Arnold, 'Official Attitudes to Population, Birth Control and Reproductive Health in India 1921–1946', in Sarah Hodges, ed. *Reproductive Health in India: History, Politics, Controversies*, New Delhi: Orient Longman, 2006, 38.

70 Mridula Ramanna, *Healthcare in Bombay Presidency, 1896–1930*, Delhi: Primus Books, 2012, see Chapter 4.

71 *Bengal Public Health Report: Reports of the Bengal Sanitary Board and the Chief Engineer Public Health Department*, Calcutta: Bengal Secretariat Book Depot, 1925.

72 Ibid.

73 Ibid.

74 Ibid.

75 'Improvement of Health: Propaganda Need', *Amrita Bazar Patrika*, 1 January 1941.

76 Fourth Health Number, *The Calcutta Municipal Gazette*, March 1932. Despite enjoying independent powers, the Corporation was subject to government intervention in the following instances: (a) In instances where implementation of a plan required a budget exceeding Rs 2.5 lakhs, local government's approval was required; (b) While the Corporation has the freedom to employ workers and pay their salaries, the appointment and pay of certain category of officials such as Chief Engineer, Health Officer etc. was subject to approval of the local government; (c) The government had the right to appoint officers to enquire into the functioning of the Corporation or to reject any decision of the Corporation that was deemed unlawful by the government. Upendranath Basu, *Kolikata o Uhar Corporation*, Second Edition, Calcutta: Sri Gouranga Press, 1944.

77 Mark Harrison has argued that the hostility between the European and the Bengali Municipal Commissioners hampered sanitary reform in the last quarter of the nineteenth century. Even the passage of the Municipal Act of 1899 which accorded primacy to the Europeans could not bring about any improvement as the hostility continued unabated. Sanitary reform was also obstructed by the cultural prejudices of the Hindu rentier class and opposed on economic grounds by the taxpayers who resented any move towards increasing local taxes for sanitary reforms. It was only after the Municipal Act of 1923 that the Hindu representation in the Corporation was once again broadened. The mortality figures remained disturbingly high at least till 1912. See Mark Harrison, *Public Health in British India: Anglo-Indian Preventive Medicine, 1859–1914*, Cambridge:

Cambridge University Press, 1995, Chapter 8. Despite the frequent clashes noted by Harrison, my research shows a broadening of activities pertaining to maternal and infant health in the years following 1912.

78  Kabita Ray has talked of Corporation's role in public health movement but has not elaborated on its important contribution towards the advancement of maternal and child welfare movement in Calcutta. Ray, *History of Public Health*. Similarly, Supriya Guha has cursorily mentioned the significance of the Corporation in producing trained midwives for domiciliary practices but has not analysed the process through which the maternal and child welfare schemes initiated by the Corporation enabled the consolidation of professional authority over childbirth. See Guha, 'Medicalisation of Childbirth'.

79  Arney, *Power and the Profession of Obstetrics*.

80  The lower middle class in the nineteenth and the twentieth centuries was largely composed of unsuccessful bhadralok. Sumit Sarkar describes them as 'pandits losing patronage in the new era, obscure hack-writers, humble school teachers, clerks, unemployed educated youth, high-school boys with highly uncertain job prospects . . . theirs has been a predominantly high-caste, yet depressed world'. See Sumit Sarkar, 'Kaliyuga, Chakri and Bhakti: Ramakrishna and His Times', in Sumit Sarkar, ed. *Writing Social History*, Delhi: Oxford University Press, 1997, 305–306. The lower middle class lived in modest neighbourhoods in Calcutta. After 1905, due to the increasing fragmentation of land and the shrinking of employment opportunities for bhadralok as English education spread to other parts of the country, the bhadralok often were reduced to the status of lower middle class. See B.B. Misra, *The Indian Middle Classes: Their Growth in Modern Times*, London, New York and Bombay: Oxford University Press, 1961, 393. In the twentieth century, particularly in the post-1939 years, the middle class 'were pushed through the borderline of gentility towards the working class' due to inflation and rising economic competition. As one noted writer observed, the percentage of indebtedness amongst the white-collar employees in Calcutta was higher than in Bombay, Delhi and Madras. See Benoy Ghosh, 'The Crisis of Bengali Gentility in Calcutta', *The Economic Weekly*, Vol.XI, Nos.26, 27 and 28, July 1957, 823. However, the most important component of lower middle class was the unemployed educated youth of Bengal who grew in number in the post-1939 period due to inflation, famine, communal riots and, eventually, partition of India. See Marcus F. Franda, 'West Bengal', in Myron Winer, ed. *State Politics in India*, Princeton, NJ: Princeton University Press, 1968. The slum dwellers who fell under the purview of the Calcutta Municipal Corporation in the 1920s, 1930s and 1940s were the urban poor who emerged as a category in the aftermath of industrial development and urbanisation of Calcutta. This category included people from rural Bengal and the Eastern and Northern part of India who came in search of employment with the rise of jute textile and coal industries and the growth of railways, dock and bank facilities. For details see Nitai Kundu, 'The Case of Kolkata, India', in UN Habitat, ed. *Global Report on Human Settlements: The Challenge of Slums*, Part IV 'Summary of City Case Studies', London: Earthscan, 2003, 195–228.

81 The appointment of midwives was part of home-visiting scheme. It was originally proposed by Dr Cook in 1907 when the Municipal authorities sought his advice on preventive schemes to reduce infant mortality. In 1908 two midwives were appointed. See 'Scheme for the Prevention of Infantile Mortality', *The Amrita Bazar Patrika*, 6 September 1918.

82 T. Fredrick Pearse, *Report of the Health Officer*, Calcutta: The Corporation Press, 1910, 47.

83 McCleary, *The Maternity and Child Welfare Movement*, 25.

84 Crake, *Report of the Health Officer*, 1913.

85 'The Nityananda Maternity Home, Navadwip', *The Amrita Bazar Patrika*, 8 December 1915.

86 Crake, *Report of the Health Officer*, 1915.

87 Crake, *Report of the Health Officer*, 1916, 30–31.

88 Crake, *Report of the Health Officer*, 1919, 45.

89 Crake, *Report of the Health Officer*, 1923, 39.

90 Ibid.

91 Ibid.

92 Crake, *Report of the Health Officer*, 1920, 49.

93 Crake, *Report of the Health Officer*, 1924, 39.

94 T.N. Majumdar, *Report of the Health Officer of Calcutta*, Calcutta: The Corporation Press, 1931.

95 Sundari Mohan Das, 'Maternal Mortality in Calcutta and Buldeodas Maternity Home', *The Calcutta Municipal Gazette*, March 1939, 614.

96 Crake, *Report of the Health Officer*, 1924.

97 Ibid., 40.

98 L.M. Biswas, *Report of the Health Officer of Calcutta*, Calcutta: The Corporation Press, 1935, 41.

99 WBSA, Local Self-Government Department, Medical Branch, File 2M-13, Proceedings 21–48, February 1925.

100 Das, 'Maternal Mortality in Calcutta'.

101 Crake, *Report of the Health Officer*, 1928.

102 David Arnold, 'Official Attitudes'.

103 *Annual Report of the All India Institute of Hygiene and Public Health* (AIIHPH) (Hereafter: *Annual Report, AIIHPH*), Calcutta: Government of India Press, 1935, 42.

104 *Annual Report, AIIHPH*, 1934, 9.

105 Ibid., 10.

106 John Farley, *To Cast Out Disease: A History of the International Health Division of the Rockefeller Foundation (1913–1951)*, New York: Oxford University Press, 2004, Chapter 15. The Rockefeller Foundation's role in India in the interwar years is particularly notable in conducting hookworm and malaria control campaigns and in setting up model rural health units. The Foundation also financed the founding of an All India College of Nursing in Delhi in 1946 in order to facilitate an increase in the number of female public health workers and nurses and also to initiate improvements in the standard of nursing profession in India. In Bengal, its most remarkable achievements were, as has been mentioned in this chapter, the foundation of the All India Institute of Hygiene and Public Health and the establishment of a chair at the School of Tropical Medicine. For more details, see Shirish N. Kavadi, *The Rockefeller*

*Foundation and Public Health in Colonial India 1916–1945: A Narrative History*, Pune and Mumbai: Foundation for Research in Community Health, 1999.

107 *Annual Report, AIIHPH*, 1935, 41.
108 Ibid.
109 Ibid.
110 S.B. Ray, 'Maternity and Child Welfare: Neglect in India, A Scheme for Calcutta Industrial Areas', *Amrita Bazar Patrika*, 11 December 1939.
111 Kavadi, *The Rockefeller Foundation*.
112 M.U. Ahmad, *Report of the Health Officer*, Calcutta: The Corporation Press, 1946–47, 7–8.
113 For instance, infant mortality in 1936 recorded an increase of 9.8 per cent over 1935. In 1937, there was a further 5.8 per cent increase over 1936 mortality figures. In 1938, however, there was a 6.7 per cent decline in the infant mortality rate. See *Bengal Public Health Report*, Alipore, Bengal: Bengal Government Press, 1936, 30; *Bengal Public Health Report*, 31; *Bengal Public Health Report*, 34.
114 *Bengal Public Health Report*, 1938, 27.
115 Majumdar, *Report of the Health Officer*, 1926, 7.
116 Kedarnath Das, P.C. Mahalanobis and Anil Chandra Nag, 'A Preliminary Note on the Rates of Maternal-Deaths and Still-Births in Calcutta', *Sankhya: The Indian Journal of Statistics*, Vol.1, No.2/3, 1935, 216–217.
117 *The Amrita Bazaar Patrika*, 9 March 1899, 4.
118 Ibid.
119 Jagjivan Basu, 'Chittaranjan Seva Sadan', *Bangalakshmi*, Vol.2, No.3, February 1927, 333–335.
120 M.I. Neal Edwards, *Report of an Enquiry into the Causes of Maternal Mortality in Calcutta*, Government of India: Manager of Publications, 1940, 34.
121 'Ramkrishna Medical College for Women: Hospital Opened by Mrs. K.C Dey', *Sunday Amrita Bazar Patrika*, 26 April 1936.
122 'Rush for Admission: Maternity Wards of Carmichael College Hospital', *Amrita Bazar Patrika*, 9 October 1936.
123 'New Maternity Ward, Howrah Hospital: Opened by Governor of Bengal', *Amrita Bazar Patrika*, 2 September 1937.
124 Samita Sen, *Women and Labour in Late Colonial India: The Bengal Jute Industry*, Cambridge: Cambridge University Press, 2004, Chapter 4.
125 *Bengal Public Health Report*, 1940.
126 Provincial legislation regulating the training and activities of midwives and nurses were passed in eight provinces such as Bihar and Orissa, Bengal, Bombay, Uttar Pradesh, Burma, Madras, Punjab and Central Provinces. The Bombay Act and that of Bihar and Orissa was passed in 1935 while those of Uttar Pradesh and Bengal were passed in 1934. For details see *Annual Report of the Public Health Commissioner with the Government of India*, Vol.I, Indian Medical Department, 1937.
127 Editorial, 'Public Health Organisation in India', *Calcutta Medical Journal*, Vol.38, No.8, August 1941, 438–441.
128 *Bengal Legislative Council Debates*, Alipore, Bengal: Bengal Government Press, 16 February 1940.

129 'Bengal Maternity Services: Deplorable State', *Amrita Bazar Patrika*, 17 April 1941.

130 Krishna Soman's ethnographic study of the Birbhum district of post-colonial Bengal shows the marginalisation of dhais in the modern health care system and their reduction to mere appendages. See Krishna Soman, 'Women, Medicine and Politics of Gender: Institution of Traditional Midwives in Twentieth Century Bengal', *Institute of Development Studies*, Occasional Paper 32, November 2011, 1–36.

131 'Maternal and Child Welfare Work: Two Lakhs Maternal Deaths a Year', *Calcutta Medical Journal*, Vol.36, No.4, October 1939, 302–304.

132 Ibid.

133 Report of the Health Survey and Development Committee, Vol.1, Delhi: Manager of Publications, 1946, Chapter 6, 64–65.

134 Arnold, 'Official Attitudes', 46.

135 Bengal Legislative Council Debates, 17 February 1945, 282.

136 Edwards, *Report of an Enquiry*, 34.

137 'Maternity and Child Welfare', *Amrita Bazar Patrika*, 12 April 1941.

# 4 The 'care-givers'

## Antenatal care in Bengali public discourse and practice, 1860s–1940s

Reviewing the progress of obstetrics in the first half of the twentieth century, R. W. Johnstone, an emeritus professor of midwifery at the University of Edinburgh, observed that of all the significant accomplishments in the domain of obstetrics such as the discovery of sulphonamides and penicillin, improvements in the methods and results of caesarean section and the triumph over puerperal fever, 'the growth of the idea of antenatal care has been the most pervasive influence, and has worked the most widespread changes in the obstetrical outlook'.[1] The main thrust of his argument:

> One line along which midwifery has been enormously improved by the antenatal idea is in the practice of the principle of physical examination of the pregnant woman from both the medical and the obstetrical points of view. Abdominal palpation of the presentation and position of the child in the later weeks of pregnancy, investigation of the capacity of the pelvis . . . routine examination of the heart and lungs . . . and the regular examination of the urine – all these are innovations of this century. The almost religious attention that is now paid to the diet of the pregnant woman is an outcome of antenatal care.[2]

The idea of antenatal care owes its origin to the redefinition of maternal and infant mortality as a 'social problem' in early twentieth-century England and other parts of Europe.[3] In Bengal, debates over the impact of maternal and infant mortality on the future of the nation and Bengali race crystallised around humanitarian, nationalist and eugenic concerns from the beginning of the twentieth century. By the end of the First World War, infant mortality was trolled in the Bengali popular print media as a potent social and national problem. Indigenous middle-class initiative was instrumental in starting a wide array of maternal and infant welfare schemes such as baby welfare shows, health exhibitions and midwifery classes which were overwhelmingly driven by the notion of 'preventability' of deaths. On a parallel plane, from 1910 onwards, the Calcutta Corporation introduced home-visiting schemes, the paramount motive being 'preservation' and 'prevention': preservation of the well-being of the expectant mother and prevent her from succumbing to diseases.

The evolution of antenatal care in Bengal was imbricated in similar developments in England, although it diverged and developed its own trajectory that was largely determined by the socio-economic realities of a colonial state. Antenatal services in Bengal were initiated by the Calcutta Corporation in 1912 in the form of home-visiting by the female health visitors attached to it. In the interwar years, the scope of antenatal care expanded owing to the mediation of voluntary bodies like the Indian Red Cross Society, Bengal Social Service League and the All India Institute of Hygiene and Public Health which started antenatal clinics in certain enclaves of Calcutta and, in the process, shared much of the burden of spreading the idea of antenatal care to Bengali women across class and religious divides.

Antenatal care was designated as 'the new midwifery' by the medical profession in the early twentieth century. In the broadest sense, antenatal care was identified with the responsibility of preserving the health of the expectant mother throughout the phase of pregnancy in order to ensure the safe delivery of a healthy child. In more strictly medical terms, it signified detection of abnormalities or illnesses during pregnancy and addressing those abnormalities through suitable and timely medical intervention. Dr J. W. Ballantyne whose claim to fame chiefly lay in the earliest espousal of the idea of antenatal care, described it as a new way of looking at old things, a 'new view point' that brought about 'momentous' changes in obstetrics practice.[4] Johnstone was also referring to a 'new outlook' in the professional growth of obstetrics that sought to extend medical control over women's bodies through 'physical examination' of her vital organs.[5]

Johnstone's prioritisation of antenatal examination of pregnant women's bodies led him to consider W. S. Playfair's popular treatise 'Science and Practice of Midwifery' (1898) as inadequate. Playfair's book was said to have lacked any direct allusion to antenatal examinations such as diagnosis of the position of the child by 'abdominal palpation', assessment of the pelvic capacity of the pregnant woman or the routine testing of her urine.[6] The fact that the textbook had 'two paragraphs' on control of constipation and 'value of proper corsetry' and also several chapters on diseases of pregnancy, meant little to

Johnstone and were, in fact, considered insufficient for removing public apathy on the value of antenatal care. In recent times, medical sociologists have equated the rise of antenatal care with the ascendancy of 'medical hegemony' over birth and the manner in which female body was slowly subjected to medical 'gaze'.[7] According to W. R. Arney, for instance, 'monitoring' of the health of the parturient woman empowered obstetrics to transcend the conventional boundaries of abnormal/pathological birth and extend its supervision over normal births as well.[8]

However, the idea of antenatal care as it evolved in colonial Bengal was predominantly about providing guidance to expectant mothers regarding preservation of health through proper diet, clothing, exercise and rest that fell more under the purview of public health administration and voluntary organisations like the Red Cross Society than medical professionals per se. Hence, it had less to do with medical hegemony being established over pregnancy and was perceived as a cheaper and yet more effective alternative to doctor-supervised hospital-based care.

Antenatal care represented the preventive side of obstetrics. The rise of 'organised preventive medicine' in England between 1875 and 1900 enabled the expansion of public health movement through sanitary reforms, supply of pure water, food, public vaccination, quarantined treatment for infectious diseases, supervision of slaughter houses and lastly a number of housing and town planning acts and factory legislation.[9] The idea of preventive medicine profoundly influenced the profession of obstetrics, especially with regard to the challenge posed by increasing rate of infant mortality. The answer was sought in antenatal care. However, systematic provision for antenatal care in England was ensured for the first time through the Local Government Board Circular issued in 1914 that underscored the State's interest in motherhood in providing medical supervision to pregnant women from conception.

More specifically, the origin and advocacy of the concept of antenatal care are usually ascribed to John William Ballantyne, a student of the University of Edinburgh and later an assistant physician at the Edinburgh Royal Maternity Hospital (1900–19) and also the president of Edinburgh Obstetrical Society. G. F. McCleary, a senior medical officer in the Ministry of Health (England) and also the principal medical officer of the National Health Insurance Commission, considered Ballantyne to be the 'greatest authority of his time on antenatal pathology, and by many is regarded as the founder of that department of medical science'.[10] Ballantyne's deepening interest in the wellbeing of the foetus encouraged him to consider whether or not it was feasible to prevent foetal abnormalities by treating the mother during pregnancy. In 1901, he pleaded for a pre-maternity hospital. In the same year, Ballantyne took over the antenatal clinic attached to the Edinburgh Royal Maternity Hospital which was then endowed with one bed (the Hamilton Bed) for the study of the diseases of pregnancy and was, henceforth, described as the 'forerunner of ante-natal ward in every modern maternity hospital'.[11] Ballantyne further contributed to the maternity and child welfare movement by publishing the first volume of 'Manual of Ante-natal Pathology and Hygiene' in 1902. In 1913, he convinced the Royal Maternity Hospital to extend its services to 'home-visiting' of expectant mothers through pre-maternity nurses attached to the hospital. In 1915, an antenatal centre was started under the supervision of the hospital called 'The Infant and Pregnancy Consultation for Expectant Mothers'. Several such antenatal clinics proliferated in the aftermath of the First World War when national anxieties over the deterioration of physical health shifted public opinion in favour of safeguarding maternal health as the first step towards ensuring the birth of healthy children.

In England, Ann Oakley has pointed out how in the first forty years of the history of evolution of antenatal care, hospital-based antenatal care was marginal as the bulk of the work was organised and provided by the municipal bodies. It was chiefly working-class women who benefitted from municipal antenatal services. The dominance of municipal authorities in providing antenatal care was enabled by the passage of the Maternity and Child Welfare Act of 1918. Within the second decade of the twentieth century, antenatal work began to progress in Australia and in the United States of America as well.[12]

## Antenatal care in Bengali popular print media in the late nineteenth century

Concerns for the health of expectant mothers emerged as part of the self-improvement drive of the western-educated Bengali middle class (bhadralok) from around the second half of the nineteenth century. Chapter 1 indicated how the western-educated bhadralok's engagement with science and modernity inspired them to embrace a rational/scientific approach to some of the vital aspects of private sphere such as domesticity, conjugality, health, motherhood, childbearing and child rearing. Midwifery and women's health figured as crucial areas of reform from the 1860s, being seen as central to the task of modernising and enlightening women. No wonder, the earliest reference to antenatal care of women during pregnancy could be noticed in print media around the same time. In a series of articles on midwifery entitled *Dhatribidya* published in *Bamabodhini Patrika* in 1867 and 1868, an essay entitled *Garbhabasthyay Prasutir Susrusa* ('Care of Pregnant Women') advised pregnant women on how to manage their own health during pregnancy. Such 'advice' literature for pregnant women came into circulation in England from the 1830s. Prominent works included P. H. Chavasse's *Advice to a Wife on the Management of her own Health* (1832) and Thomas Bull's *Hints to Mothers for the Management of Health during the Period of Pregnancy and in the Lying-in Room* (1837).[13] The instructions given to the expectant mother in the advice manuals of nineteenth-century England influenced the early Bengali writings on antenatal care.

The essay *Garbhabasthyay Prasutir Susrusa* (1867) represented one of the earliest attempts to explain the impact of maternal health on the survival of the foetus. It emphatically stated that in

> the improvement of the mother's health lies the improvement of the foetus, in her distress lies its distress, in her strength lies its strength, her nutrition nourishes the foetus, her blood sustains it, her life nurtures its life, her death therefore cannot keep the foetus alive for a long time . . . such is the connection of the mother with her child.[14]

Like the advice manuals of nineteenth-century England, the essay was devoid of technical terms. Also lacking any direct allusion to the need for medical supervision of the expectant mother, the essay was a lucid exposition of certain rational principles that an expectant mother was advised to follow in order to ensure safe delivery of the child. It insisted on proper clothing, diet, and intake of fresh air, physical exercise and the importance of sound mental health during pregnancy. It advised wearing of loose garments in order to facilitate unimpeded supply of blood to the foetus. In addition, nutritious and easily digestible food was recommended. Indigestion and intestinal complications arising out of consumption of spicy food were felt to jeopardise the life of the foetus. In this connection, the essay approved of the celebration of the age-old Bengali custom of *saadh* on a certain auspicious day in the ninth month of pregnancy. *Saadh* was celebrated with the intent of pampering the palate of the expectant mother with a choice of her favourite delicacies a few days prior to the onset of labour.

Yet another interesting article that appeared in 1892 in the women's magazine *Paricarika* dwelt on care of women during pregnancy by stating that the psychological and physical state of the mother nurtured the body and mind of the child. Pregnancy, according to this article, had always been dreaded as the time of 'thousand dangers'. Anticipating such dangers, pregnant women were advised to adopt certain precautionary measures in terms of diet, bath, exercise and rest. There was, however, no mention of the diseases associated with pregnancy.[15] The overarching theme was preservation of the general health of the expectant mother which was deemed crucial for the well-being of the foetus. Such writings were largely non-medical in approach and content. They did not overtly insist on medical supervision and physical examinations of the expectant mothers.

However, advice manuals for the care of pregnant women were few and far between in the nineteenth century. Reference to antenatal care of pregnant women was absent in Annada Charan Khastagir's seminal work, *Manabjanmatattva, Dhatribidya, Nabaprasut Sisu o Strijatir Byadhi Sangraha* ('A Treatise on the Science and Practice of Midwifery with Diseases of Women and Children') published in 1868. Similarly, in the whole new genre of literature on infant rearing that came into circulation in the late nineteenth century, discussions on antenatal care found only sporadic mention. Essays on postnatal care of women under such titles as *Anturghar e Prasutir Susrusa* ('Care of the Mother after Childbirth') were, however, more frequently published and continued to appear, from time to time, in *Bamabodhini Patrika*, *Bharati* and *Antahpur*. They chiefly consisted of instructions on proper diet of the mother soon after delivery, on hygiene, cleanliness and tips on infant feeding including breastfeeding.

Scientific treatises on midwifery, composed by male licentiate doctors in Bengali language, began to be published in the 1870s and 1880s. While such textbooks mostly lacked any direct allusion to antenatal care, Haranath Ray's *Dhatri-siksha Samgraha* ('Midwife's Vade-Mecum') published in 1887 contained an elaborate section on the diet of pregnant women under the title *Garbhinir pathya o svasthya vijnan* ('Diet of Pregnant Women and Health Science'). Basing his argument on the research findings in European laboratories, Ray stated that the diet of pregnant women should be free of 'earthy' and 'bony' substances which were likely to harden the pelvic region and obstruct the smooth passage of the child during delivery. Ray proscribed the consumption of wheat, meat, dairy products and excessive salt. Instead a balanced diet of vegetables and fruits suiting Bengali conditions was recommended and 'distilled' water was prioritised over tap water. Drawing on his reading of Thomas Bull's advice manual, Ray discarded the age-old belief that overfeeding of the expectant mother provided nourishment to the foetus. He also denounced the custom of *saadh* which, in his opinion, could damage the health of the expectant mother by causing vomiting, digestive ailments and constipation. Ray prescribed daily bathing in cold water which would soften the perineum and alleviate breast pain. He finally argued, 'It is undoubted that pain during labour is a part of the process and hence an act of nature. However, it is also logical to make sure that labour itself should not become protracted and painful.'[16] Ray's comment thus vaguely alluded to the 'preventive' side of obstetrics and the way it could avert any possible danger during labour.

## Antenatal care in the nationalist discourse

At the turn of the century, the idea of preventive medicine influenced the Bengali medical profession in analysing public health problems. In this context, it is cogent to quote the objectives of a prominent health magazine *Svasthya Samachar* as vividly outlined by the editor Dr Kartikchandra Basu in its inaugural issue published in 1912. It stated:

> The domain of health is vast and with the advancement of science, it is also acquiring progress with each passing day. In contemporary Europe and America, preventive medicine is being extensively discussed as an important branch of medical science and is being taught to the lay public through easily readable books, contemporary newspapers and lectures. Our country also has a rich tradition of . . . treatments initiated by Caraka, Susruta and other illustrious medical men, but they have barely been disseminated to the general public. Most of them are confined to the books. On the other hand, with the progress of time, there has been a lot of transformation in our country. The arrangements put in place three thousand years ago by the wise Aryan hermits of the Himachal are not easily attainable by the civilised people of the 20th century . . . Hence, this magazine is published with the aim to ensure that the basic principles of health management and means to resist disease founded on an awareness of the Eastern and Western medical principles should reach a wider reading public so as to enable them to safeguard their health as well as the health of others. This magazine, will therefore, publish extensive discussions on discoveries of new theories and facts about health in different parts of the world.[17]

Here the author's insistence on the importance of 'preventive medicine' was an echo of the international medical opinion promoting its
centrality in reducing mortality rates. In the years following 1914,
western medical science and technology in bhadralok imagination
were no longer directly associated with the colonial structure per se
but instead came to be identified with modernity and the reconfiguration of the emerging nation.[18] Quite predictably therefore, *Svasthya
Samachar* which essentially targeted the middle-class readership in
Bengal reflected a commitment towards broadening the horizon of
the readers through publishing national and international accomplishments in medical research and discoveries. It was this growing cosmopolitanism that shaped the outlook of the Bengali medical profession
towards pregnancy and childbirth as reflected in the textual spaces of
the health magazines.

In England, at the turn of the century, antenatal care was considered
a vital part of preventive obstetrics. Eugenics broadly defined as the
'well-being of the race' provided a powerful context for recognising
'the value of the *potential* mother and her *unborn babe* as a *national
asset*' (emphasis mine).[19] One of the broader purposes of eugenics
was prevention of the birth of 'weaklings' and 'unfit' children. Antenatal care, in this sense, was expected to prevent the 'extermination'
of babies and ensure a process of rectification of 'unfitness' through
'ameliorating' it antenatally. The spotlight was hence on 'antenatal'
pathology. It was argued that

> ante-natal pathology being the subject which deals with foetal dis-
> eases, embryonic deformities . . . must play an important part in
> any attempt to ensure ante-natal hygiene. To prevent the produc-
> tion of the unfit it is manifestly necessary that we learn the causes
> of their unfitness and their mode of action.[20]

Thus, the necessity to 'unravel the pathological mysteries' of diseases associated with pregnancy was beginning to be perceived as an
important social and medical obligation of the medical profession
from a eugenic standpoint. To cite an instance, eugenic considerations inspired one Dr Amand Routh of the Charing Cross Hospital in
London to undertake an investigation into the nature of 'toxaemias'
during pregnancy in 1911.[21] Such ideas echoed in the writings of
Bengali medical men as well.[22]

Publications on antenatal care in Bengali popular print remained
few in the early decades of the twentieth century. Concerns for health

of the infant as the foundation of a strong Bengali race drew cogent connections between maternal health and infant mortality. Early twentieth-century popular health magazines addressed such concerns by highlighting the debilitating impact of maternal diseases on infant health. Consequently, maternal diseases or diseases associated with pregnancy became an integral component of the discussion on ante-natal care. To cite an example, an article entitled *Garbhinir Kartabya* ('Duties of a Pregnant Woman') published in *Svasthya Samachar* in 1916 marked a subtle departure from the nineteenth-century writings in its emphasis on pathologies associated with pregnancy and the importance of prior medical consultation in averting infant mortality and damage to the unborn foetus. It explained the possibility of infants inheriting physical weakness from their mothers who might have been afflicted with liver ailments or respiratory troubles during pregnancy. It provided hints on heart ailments and symptoms of kidney diseases such as swelling of feet that could surface during pregnancy and endanger the life of the foetus. It also highlighted the importance of medical intervention in correcting 'pelvic deformities'. The article also urged Bengali women to shed their modesty for the greater benefit of the unborn child and seek the assistance of a doctor in cases of illness.[23] The most perceptible feature of the article was, therefore, its insistence on medical consultation.

The need to guide the expectant mother during the puerperal period continued to be articulated in Bengali health journals throughout the second decade of the twentieth century. The elderly women of the household, the 'experienced' mother-in law in particular, were appreciated for guiding the young daughter-in law on the commencement of her pregnancy through a careful selection of her diet, domestic work and watching her physical movement within the household and contact with her husband. Young expectant mothers were admonished for their reluctance to adhere to health rules. European women were idealised as the bearers of modernity and lauded for their commitment to a disciplined and healthy lifestyle. Like her European counterpart, the Bengali woman had to be aware of the importance of protecting the foetus in its 'pre-natal existence'.[24]

At the peak of nationalist movement in the 1920s and 1930s, western scientific knowledge was often disseminated by emphasising its similarities with the indigenous medical traditions. Such propensities were evident in the writings of Bengali medical professionals. An example of this trend is Girindra Krishna Mitra's *Prasuti o Santan* ('Pregnant Woman and the Infant') published in 1929. Having received his higher education in Dublin, Mitra was inspired by the progress of antenatal care in the United Kingdom and in other western countries and liberally drew upon the works of Truby King and F. J. Browne.[25] Yet being aware of the force of nationalism in the cultural discourse of the Bengalis, he carefully couched his argument in nationalist terms.[26]

Mitra's text was grounded in welding western medical discourse and the Ayurveda tradition – redefined as 'national' in the phase of anticolonial struggle – within a cohesive explanatory framework. Scholars have argued how attempts to impart professional and scientific status to Ayurveda was an essential component of the nationalisation of indigenous medical tradition; it perhaps pointed to the process by which a national cultural identity was carved out during the heights of national movement in colonial India.[27] Thus, Mitra's text underscored the importance of routine physical examination of women during pregnancy by referring to the existence of similar prescriptions in Caraka's Ayurvedic formulations 2,500 years ago. It indicated how Caraka's Ayurvedic treatise contained a section on care of pregnant women in matters of diet, clothing and general health. Mitra's text also referred to the minor diseases of pregnancy such as constipation, nausea, indigestion, swelling of feet, skin diseases and major problems like eclampsia and presence of albumin in urine. It explained the importance of examination of urine in order to detect the presence of albumin and advised medical consultation in case of albumin being found in urine. The text also prescribed the appointment of a midwife or physician immediately after conception (*garbhadhan*). The moot point was as follows:

> Pregnancy is a natural process, but it *demands adequate medical supervision*. The health of the mother and the child within depends a lot on proper nurturing. The pressure is mostly on liver, kidney, heart and other organs for the nutrition and sustenance of the foetus . . . if one of the organs stops functioning properly, it harms the health of the mother and hence weakens the foetus. If proper care is taken, 90% of the mothers can be liberated from diseases and hence, can give birth to healthy and strong children. (emphasis mine)[28]

The middle-class women groups in Bengal too argued in favour of medical supervision during pregnancy. Magazines like *Bangalakshmi*, which was published from the 1920s, assumed a central role in articulating middle-class feminist consciousness in Bengal. *Bangalakshmi* contained instructive essays on care of pregnant women. One such essay entitled *Garbhinir Gyatabya* ('Things an Expectant Mother Should Know') began with the assertion:

> Pregnancy and Childbirth are the two most defining events in a woman's life. In this state, there is danger at every step. Hence, it is important to be careful and cautious. It is important to know the rules that should be followed during pregnancy, especially by women themselves, but that does not mean that doctor or midwife should not be consulted at all.

The essay prescribed proper course of diet and bath for pregnant women, also advising extra precautionary measures in the last three months of pregnancy.[29]

Baby shows became a regular medium through which antenatal and postnatal advices on maternal health and infant rearing were disseminated to the mothers, although its popularity was questionable at all times. At the All India Baby Week Conference held in Calcutta in 1924, Dr V. B. Green-Armytage, the professor of midwifery and gynaecology at the CMC, explained the importance of antenatal care as the 'new midwifery' in obstetric practice. Green-Armytage redefined the instrumentality of an event like baby week in promoting antenatal care in the following words:

> The title *Baby Week* infers a greater item, namely *babies before birth*, for we must do something radical to stem the fearsome maternal and child mortality and morbidity in India, and this *something* is what is designated as the *new midwifery*. It is no use catering alone for the sick child after it is sick, or after it has been born into the world of a sickly mother – your baby clinics do that and do it well; but what we must do, is to develop a far, more important scheme, that of *antenatal care*. (emphasis original)[30]

At the Baby Week Conference, Green-Armytage distributed a diagram of the female anatomy in parturient state which he had drawn with the assistance of the Baptist Mission Press. Entitled 'A Scheme of Enquiry for the Prevention of Troubles in the Expectant Mother and Neo-Natal Infant', the diagram was a detailed exposition of the various illnesses associated with pregnancy. It was intended to guide the training of voluntary health workers whom Green-Armytage termed female 'Sherlock Holmes' whose duties were to assume the role of 'sleuth-hounds' in locating and preventing diseases and accidents during pregnancy. Further, with the help of the diagram Green-Armytage demonstrated how the antenatal detection of contracted pelvis of the expectant mother at an early stage of pregnancy was crucial in deciding upon a timely caesarean section which could save both maternal and infant life. The purpose of antenatal care was also to discover a history of difficult labour or miscarriage and find out whether the baby was a breech instead of being a head presentation.[31]

Green-Armytage advocated propaganda, efficient training of the female health workers and cooperation between the female health workers and the doctors as the three chief ways to assist the Bengali mothers in shedding inhibitions and seeking medical care during pregnancy. Towards the end of the 1920s, Green-Armytage went on to incorporate a chapter on antenatal care and also an antenatal chart in the appendix in his popular textbook for medical students entitled *Tropical Midwifery: Labour Room Clinics*, which was published in 1928.[32] The central theme of the chapter was diet of the pregnant women which according to him was 'of immense importance in the prevention of disease in both mother and child'.[33]

From the 1940s, Bengali medical professionals utilised nationalist press as a platform to publicise the idea of antenatal care by citing eugenic concerns and national welfare. Dr Subodh Mitra wrote in *Amrita Bazar Patrika*, 'If prevention is supposed to be the best remedy, it should be instituted at the very root, and thus a system of "constructive" hygiene may be developed for the raising of a new generation.'[34] Thus, 'proper' diet, clothing and hygiene for pregnant women were prioritised while the tendencies to eliminate abnormalities by operative interference were denounced. It was argued that the 'obstetrician should not seek recognition or praise for the dexterity with which he has interfered'.[35]

The economic constraints of Bengal administration were amply recognised by the Public Health officials in arguing for cheaper antenatal and postnatal services for pregnant women. In this connection, A. C. Chatterjee, the director of Public Health in Bengal argued in 1941 that:

> It is far more desirable and economical if the vast majority of normal labour cases could be delivered at home. Pregnancy is a normal physiological function of a woman and *if proper health education is imparted to every woman and adequate antenatal attention could be given to the expectant mothers there should be no difficulty in her going through the experience in her own home, in which case only domiciliary midwifery services may be required* . . . maternity homes and maternity hospitals are

necessary but they should be more in the form of insurance rather than as a place where every pregnant woman should go as a matter of routine for delivering her child.(emphasis mine)[36]

The focus was therefore on a scheme in which the bulk of 'normal' deliveries would ideally take place at homes under the guidance of health visitors and trained midwives while only complicated cases would be 'timely' shifted to the hospitals.

Other medical professionals also shared similar views. Dr Gorachand Nandi, a deputy visiting surgeon at the Chittaranjan Seva Sadan Hospital, read a paper at the Calcutta Medical Club in 1941 stating that while adequate antenatal care could entail considerable expenditure, it could also curtail expenses in other directions. It would not only 'enormously' reduce the number of septic beds that were invariably also the most expensive ones, but also minimise the number of beds allocated for gynaecological complications and operations arising out of infection or injury caused by childbirth due to the absence of antenatal supervision during pregnancy. Such beds were a burden on the government and public hospitals. Like Subodh Mitra, Nandi also denounced unnecessary operative interference following antenatal supervisions stating that it 'does not help a woman very much if she is rescued from the hypothetical consequences of an abnormality and is killed in effecting a rescue'.[37]

Although operative interventions were discouraged and cheaper ways of providing antenatal care were being argued for, a benign form of medical supervision of the pregnant woman's health through antenatal examinations such as urine test, blood pressure and measurements of the pelvis was beginning to be suggested in the interwar years.[38] From the 1930s, however, preventive obstetrics and medical supervision acquired centrality in the discourse on maternal and infant welfare in India.

## Diseases in pregnancy and preventive obstetrics

Research on the preventable aspects of maternal and infant mortality became a national and political imperative in England from the 1920s. The 1920s had witnessed noticeable improvements in the sphere of maternal and child health, the most significant being the formation of the Ministry of Health in 1919 that took over the administration of maternal and child welfare–related issues. In 1924, the first comprehensive government report on maternal mortality was published that was written by Janet Campbell, Senior Medical Officer to the department administering maternal and child welfare within the Ministry of Health. While highlighting the causes of maternal mortality to be improper professional attendance, abortions, rickets and specific diseases like sepsis, toxaemias and haemorrhage, Campbell's report also focused extensively on the preventive aspects of obstetrics. Arguing that most of the deaths or illnesses associated with pregnancy were 'avoidable', the report reiterated the centrality of antenatal supervision in the reduction of maternal mortality. It was stated that all attempts to curb maternal and infant mortality and promote improvement in the conditions of childbirth would be rendered futile if mothers did not realise the importance of placing themselves under medical guidance from the onset of pregnancy. It was equally important for the doctors and the midwives to realise the worth of antenatal supervision in saving lives.[39]

Campbell's report was analysed with regard to Indian conditions by Dr Margaret Balfour. Balfour's report was subsequently published in the *Indian Medical Gazette* in December 1924. Balfour commented that despite the absence of a Maternity and Child Welfare Act in India like the one passed in England or the lack of initiatives from the local bodies, antenatal work could still be conducted by every medical practitioner by forming his/her own antenatal centre connected with the consulting room. Balfour further argued that Indian doctors and midwives had to lay the foundations of antenatal work which would then be embraced by the local bodies.[40]

Investigations into the causes of maternal mortality began to be conducted in India in the 1920s under the institutional guidance of the Indian Research Fund Association which came into being in 1911 and was funded by the Government of India.[41] In analysing maternal morbidity in India, such researches identified the diseases in pregnancy and, in the process, redefined birth as a pathological condition requiring medical supervision. However, lack of reliable mortality figures attributed to 'defective' birth registrations and failure of large maternity hospitals to preserve records of births and deaths constituted serious constraints in collating data for research purposes.

An initial enquiry on the causes of maternal mortality in India was conducted by the Indian Research Fund Association in 1925. The findings were later published in a report entitled, 'Maternal Mortality in Childbirth in India'.[42] The investigation was based on questionnaires sent out to all the major maternity wards and hospitals in India. The data received were classified and compared to similar figures for hospitals in England and Ireland. The significance of the report lay in its in-depth analysis of the diseases of pregnancy that were shown to substantially affect the maternal mortality figures in India. The report stated:

> There has been a general impression for many years past that the conditions of childbirth in India are difficult and the mortality high; this has been popularly put down to the wretched attendance for women at the time of childbirth, and to the lack of medical relief when necessary, but those who have seen much of obstetrics have been aware that there is also much disease in pregnancy.[43]

It identified several diseases during pregnancy such as anaemia, eclampsia, osteomalacia, venereal diseases, 'accidents or complications during pregnancy or labour' and 'size of pelvis'. It concluded that there was 'much disease connected with pregnancy in India' that was squarely responsible for the 'greater part' of maternal mortality, stillbirths and infant mortality. The remedy was sought in antenatal care. The research concluded by highlighting the importance of antenatal research.[44]

From the 1920s female medical professionals associated with the Women Medical Service (WMS), established in India in 1912, undertook researches into the causes of maternal mortality in India that were funded by the Indian Research Fund Association. At the Far Eastern Association of Tropical Medical Congress in 1927, Margaret Balfour read a paper on the factors affecting maternal mortality in India. She identified anaemia, eclampsia and osteomalacia as the chief causes of maternal mortality in the country. Agnes Scott's paper, also read at the Congress, was yet another detailed analysis of the geographical variation in the incidence of osteomalacia.[45] In the 1930s, the medical women attached to the newly established All India Institute of Hygiene and Public Health (AIIHPH) in Calcutta sought the cooperation of the Health Officer of the Corporation in carrying out studies on 'pyorrhoea' during pregnancy or on the impact of nutrition on maternal and infant health.[46]

On another plane, the centrality of pelvic measurement in ascertaining the normal/abnormal character of pregnancy stimulated obstetric research on the size of pelvis of Indian women. Critical enquiry into the 'relation of childbearing to the progressive development of the female pelvis' came to be carried out by medical men from the second decade of the twentieth century.[47] Dr Grace Stapleton's study of pelvic measurements of Indian women in the city of Agra in 1925 constituted one such effort.[48] In a similar vein, Kathleen Vaughan's research in Kashmir showed how pregnancy was a perfectly normal function when the pelvis fitted the size of the foetal head. According to Vaughan, contracted pelvis that impeded smooth passage of foetal head during labour was a consequence of rickets, prolonged confinement in the zenana and lack of manual labour.[49]

However, it was the trope of purdah that emerged as the most identifiable source of diseases causing contraction of pelvis. In 1929 Hemangini Sen, the editor of *Bangalakshmi*, critiqued the insanitary conditions of Bengali homes that, according to her, were shut off from sunlight and fresh air and, hence, caused respiratory and heart diseases amongst Bengali females. Sen therefore singled out purdah as the most potent source of disease.[50] Similarly Kathleen Vaughan, in one of her earlier work, had attributed osteomalacia or the softening of bones amongst Kashmiri women to the observance of purdah and in the process overlooked other plausible causes such as deficient diet. The use of purdah as a trope was later evident in the Indian feminist discourse that sought to associate it with maternal morbidity, birth of weaklings and the consequent moral and physical degeneration of the Indian race.[51] In this connection, Maneesha Lal has argued that western medical discourse's overemphasis on purdah as the most potent source of female diseases led to other socio-economic factors perpetuating women's ill health such as poverty, overcrowding, malnutrition, colonial socio-economic policies and patriarchal dominations being ignored and marginalised.[52]

In 1929, the Departmental Committee on Maternal Mortality and Morbidity under the Ministry of Health of England issued a Memorandum defining the scope of antenatal care in England. It was entitled 'Antenatal Clinics: Their Conduct and Scope'.[53] This was followed by two reports on maternal mortality and morbidity issued in 1930 and 1932 by the same committee. In these reports, 49 per cent of the maternal deaths were considered to be preventable, while 17 per cent of them were attributed to the absence of antenatal care. It was also estimated that the rate of stillbirths would fall by 50 per cent if adequate antenatal care was provided to the pregnant women. The findings of the report were analysed in the *Calcutta Medical Journal* and in the Bengali magazine *Byabosa O Banijya*, the sole purpose being to reiterate the 'preventability' of maternal deaths during childbirth.[54] The annual reports of the All India Institute of Hygiene and Public Health also confirmed that most of the maternal deaths in Calcutta were preventable.[55]

Diet of the expectant mother also became an intense area of research funded by the Countess of Dufferin Fund and the Indian Research Fund Association. Efforts to standardise the diet of pregnant women along established standards of nutrition constituted the chief focus of such research. It encouraged further probes into the causes of 'deficiency' diseases that were stated to arise out of 'ill-balanced' diet or lack of vitamins.[56] Also the occurrence of pregnancy-related anaemia was linked to the dietary and hygienic habits of the Bengalis in Calcutta.[57]

Thus, researches into causes of maternal mortality in India in the early decades of the twentieth century brought forth the diseases associated with pregnancy and explained the need to diagnose and cure them antenatally through medical supervision and intervention when appropriate. Such assertions became fundamental to the professionalisation of obstetrics in Bengal in the interwar years. Dr G. G. Jolly of the IMS had stated in 1940:

> Each stage prenatal, natal and postnatal may with luck be safely negotiated without the aid of doctor or nurse, but it is a proved fact that mother stands the best chance of safe delivery and a healthy child who obtains and follows expert medical advice throughout. Much responsibility can and in most cases must be devolved upon health visitors and midwives, but our efforts should be directed towards securing the minimum necessary examination and supervision by a qualified doctor in every case.[58]

Yet, in the specific socio-economic context of Bengal, antenatal care was understood by the public health officials and some medical professionals as ideally an inexpensive and affordable alternative to doctor-supervised hospital-based birth. All attempts were directed towards promoting home-birth under the care of trained midwives or health visitors.

## The care-givers in action, 1912–1947

A close study of the antenatal work undertaken in Bengal in the late colonial period reveals the predominance of the public health workers, municipalities and voluntary bodies and the marginality of institution/hospital-based endeavours. In 1912, when new regulations for the MB degree were introduced by the Calcutta University, special instructions in antenatal care and infant hygiene were made mandatory for the candidates.[59] That was indeed a major step towards including antenatal care as an important element of obstetrics. Yet, antenatal services were initiated by the Calcutta Municipal Corporation and not by the CMC. By 1912, the Corporation had already formulated schemes to provide health care to pregnant women in the form of home-visiting, although the focus was primarily on lower-middle-class and poor mothers.

Home-visiting was started in 1912 by a newly evolved category of female health visitor previously designated as sanitary inspector. In the same year, the female health visitor was reported to have spoken to 200 pregnant women and advised them in 82 cases to seek the care of corporation midwives. The Health Visitor also stated in her report how detection of anaemia during pregnancy in the course of home-visiting led to the delivery of the pregnant women at the hospital and in the process saved her life.[60] Within two years, the annual report of the Corporation recorded the increase in the number of home-visits by leaps and bounds. In 1914 a single lady health visitor was reported to have 'visited 3, 666 homes in which 6,740 families were living; no fewer than 6,740 women were interviewed and given simple instructions chiefly in the care and management of children. Largely owing to the excellent relations established with the *dhais*, 545 newly-born babies were visited'.[61]

A chain of maternity centres established by the Corporation in the 1920s brought into being a scheme of domiciliary midwifery services sustained by a staff of female health visitors and trained midwives. The domiciliary midwifery service enabled the management of normal delivery at home while transferring difficult or complicated cases to the hospital and maternity homes run by the Corporation. The trend continued in the subsequent decades. Despite remarkable increase in home-visiting, the recalcitrance of the allegedly 'prejudiced' and 'ignorant' slum dwellers was often a serious obstacle recounted in such reports. Thus, one Miss Lewis recounted how, 'the *bustee* (slum) people were afraid and hid their women if they were pregnant and gave us no information or help'.[62]

Postnatal care constituted a more significant part of Corporation's work. In 1916, a scheme of visiting the babies delivered by municipal midwives was introduced as a form of postnatal supervision. The difficulty of convincing mothers to bring their babies to the hospitals for postnatal check-up led to home-visiting being deemed as the only viable alternative. Thus, it was laid down that as soon as the puerperal period of ten days was over, the babies would be entered into the registers of the female health visitors whose principal task would be to pay home-visits and systematically monitor the health of the baby up to three months after birth on a weekly or fortnightly basis. Although the progress of the baby welfare work was reported to be slow in the absence of adequate health visitors, provisions were still made for the supervision of the poor mother and her child. This included providing 'nourishing food' for the mother, milk for the baby, warm clothing for the infants to brave the winters and also medicines such as ergot, quinine and castor oil.[63] By 1920, there were four maternity centres conducting home-visiting and deliveries of pregnant women. Three more child welfare centres for postnatal and baby welfare purposes were added to the existing system in 1921.[64]

The question of milk supply became integral to postnatal work. As early as in 1908, the Corporation was praised for its laudable effort to build sanitary cowsheds and prevent adulteration of milk as a veritable panacea for infant mortality.[65] In 1915, J. Patson, the Assistant Director of Dairy Farms, was appointed by the government to inquire into the problems related to pure milk supply in Calcutta. Amongst his recommendations, the important ones were for the establishment of Calcutta Corporation dairy farm and further investigations into the quality of milk produced in the mufassils. The Health Officer of the Corporation further articulated in 1916 the urgent need of 'municipalising' milk supply for the whole of the city of Calcutta. Aid from the affluent sections of the society was deemed essential in establishing milk depots in every part of the city and in ensuring the preparation and supply of 'humanised' milk at a low price for the purpose of feeding the infants. In 1921, the first step was taken in this direction by the establishment of five baby clinics and milk depots in different parts of Calcutta by the Indian National Association and the St. Johns Ambulance Association. The milk kitchens attached to the clinics supplied free milk to the infants.

Doubts on the efficacy of the Corporation schemes in ensuring pure milk supply were expressed in the media from time to time. Such debates were subsumed within a larger and more complex political drive for cow protection that hinged on the logic that cultivation of land was dependent on cattles; the thoughtless killing of cows by the Muslims steadily contributed towards a declining agriculture and dwindling economy.[66] Creative measures such as importing cows from abroad and maintaining them in 'model sheds' in the suburbs of Calcutta were also suggested.[67] In 1924 the Corporation opened six milk kitchens and child welfare centres and placed them under the control of a trained nurse. The milk kitchens were reconstituted and increased in number in 1934 to ensure free supply of milk to greater number of babies below two years of age and, later on, to women's welfare organisations such as the *Hindu Nari Kalyan Ashram* (Hindu women welfare society), *Hindu Abala Ashram* (Abode for Helpless Hindu

Women), *Bengal Social Service League* etc. The total number of babies registered in the milk kitchens showed a steady rise in the late 1920s and 1930s.[68]

Eradication of maternal ignorance emerged as one of the key planks in the promotion and expansion of preventive obstetrics in the inter-war years. At a time when the educative aspects of antenatal care were being emphasised by medical men, public health officials and the Bengali press, the Calcutta Corporation took up the significant task of enlightening mothers on health and hygiene from 1912. In 1914, the first female health visitor remarked, 'As education spreads, the need and opportunity for instructing wives and mothers in the principles of public and domestic hygiene increase. Even educated lady, not to speak of the half-educated and the illiterate, have exceedingly vague ideas of hygienic principles.'[69] From 1912 onwards, mothers were given instruction in elementary hygiene and infant feeding during home-visits. From the 1920s, education of mothers was incorporated into the work of the baby welfare clinics.

The early history of the evolution of antenatal services in Bengal was, therefore, dominated by home-visiting facilities provided by the Calcutta Corporation and the provincial municipalities, the most noteworthy being those in Darjeeling, Dacca, Rangpur and Rajshahi. From 1915, the Bengal Social Service League, a voluntary organisation, contributed significantly towards maternal and infant welfare work. Its chief contribution lay in establishing a maternity and infant welfare centre in a 'Settlement house' which was built on a gift of land from the Calcutta Corporation and was located in a Muslim-dominated '*bustee*' area (slum) in the northern part of Calcutta. The League offered to Muslim women mother-craft lessons that included antenatal advice on diet and general health care during pregnancy. The European health visitor, Luise Gompertz, who was in charge of the Settlement House recounted in the 1940s that the mothers who adhered to such advices during pregnancy often recovered 'most wonderfully' from illness and on a daily dose of milk, iron, calcium and cod-liver oil regained strength by the time their babies arrived.[70] By the 1930s, there were twenty-two maternity and infant welfare clinics outside Calcutta, where pregnant women were registered and provided antenatal care, apart from home-visits being made by health visitors when necessary. Abnormal cases were transferred to the hospitals.[71] However, antenatal work did not figure prominently in the expanding domain of activities of the Saroj Nalini Dutt Memorial Association (SNDMA) which was entirely managed by middle-class

Bengali women and contributed significantly to the starting of *dhai* training classes, mother-craft lessons and establishment of baby clinics in the districts of Bengal.[72]

The foundation of the All India Institute of Hygiene and Public Health (AIIHPH) in 1934 and the Bengal Health Welfare Committee under the Indian Red Cross Society in 1936 expanded the ambit of antenatal work in Calcutta and the outlying areas. The AIIHPH, as mentioned in Chapter 3, was a major institutional site for the training of public health workers including maternity and child welfare workers. In 1935, the institute established a maternity and child welfare centre in Ward 8, located in the north-central part of the city that housed antenatal, infant and toddler clinics. Within a year of the establishment of the antenatal clinic, an attendance of 54 per cent out of a total of 384 cases identified was recorded in the annual report of the institute.[73] It showed a steady growth in the subsequent years. However, the 1938 annual report showed that only 26.5 per cent of women attending the clinic received 'complete' antenatal, intranatal and postnatal care. That included two visits by pregnant women to the centre, monthly domiciliary advice by health visitor, delivery of child by the midwife attached to the institution and, lastly, postnatal care by the midwife, health visitor and the doctor; 18.2 per cent of the women had delivery at hospitals and maternity homes, 10.9 per cent by other midwives, 1.9 per cent by private doctors and, lastly, 43.1 per cent by untrained dhais.[74] The report therefore revealed the inconsistencies in the antenatal work conducted in Calcutta that resulted in actual care being restricted to the puerperal period while most of the deliveries continued to be managed by dhais and relatives of the mother. Consequently, most of the pregnant women attending the antenatal clinic remained outside direct medical supervision.

Yet, the work of the maternity and child welfare centre attached to the AIIHPH served as a model for the Red Cross Society in establishing its sphere of activities in Bengal. The results achieved by the maternity and child welfare centre under AIIHPH 'were found to be so good it was thought the Red Cross could do no better than follow the excellent example there presented'.[75] Consequently the Bengal Health Welfare Committee (BHWC) was established as a voluntary body in 1936. Under the revised plan of the newly formed BHWC, each of the six maternity and child welfare centres under its control was to operate within a limited area, providing health service to all expectant mothers and to those with newborn babies and infants within its jurisdiction. The maternity benefit scheme launched by the Committee was composed of six committees: 'Calcutta Maternity and Child

Welfare Committee', 'District Maternity and Child Welfare Committee', 'Industrial Welfare Committee', 'Bengal Health Education Committee', 'Calcutta Health Week Committee' and 'Sir John Anderson Health School'. Calcutta and the outlying mufassils and districts formed the area of activities of these committees.[76]

BHWC's contribution to maternity and child welfare work chiefly lay in instituting antenatal work in the areas surrounding the maternity and child welfare centres run by it. There were six maternity centres, chiefly the Entally Centre, Kidderpore Centre, Bhowanipore Centre, the Northern Centre and later on a *Shasthya Niketan* Centre (which replaced the Bhowanipore centre) and, lastly, Servants of Humanity Society in Suhrawardy Avenue. Antenatal care was provided in the form of home-visits and attendance of expectant mothers in the antenatal clinics attached to the maternity centres. The antenatal clinics were reported to have made 'thorough routine examination of each case' including urine test, estimation of blood pressure and haemoglobin percentage. Prescription on diet, instructions on hygiene and simple treatment for anaemia, calcium deficiency also constituted important tasks of the clinics. Abnormal or serious cases were moved to the hospital. Mother-craft classes conducted throughout the year also formed a part of the routine of the maternity and child welfare centres of the BHWC.

However, the BHWC complained of poverty and purdah system as the chief sociocultural constraints that prevented pregnant women from seeking antenatal care. For instance, in the area surrounding the Entally Centre which was largely inhabited by the Muslim population, antenatal work was stated to be obstructed by the purdah system. It was pointed out that the practice of seclusion prevented Muslim women from attending the antenatal clinics and also from going to the hospital even when seriously ill. Consequently, in the first annual report of the BHWC, the Entally Centre was shown to have displayed the 'lowest attendance at the clinics and the highest mortality rates'. The reason for the failure was 'not due to lack of energy and enthusiasm on the part of the workers but to the difficult nature of the population'.[77] A similar situation was noted for the Kidderpore Centre which too was located in a predominantly Muslim neighbourhood.

It is difficult to ascertain from the existing sources the percentage of Bengali middle-class women willingly placing themselves under the antenatal care provided by the clinics. Dr Ruth Young complained till the late 1920s about the reluctance of Indian women in appreciating the worth of antenatal care, an attitude that derived considerable support from the elderly female members of the joint family. Young further pointed out that

> in the middle classes it is often impossible for a young woman in this state even to go out. It is not considered proper and the latter part of pregnancy has to be spent within the home. Among the poorer and the labouring classes the latter objection may not hold good, but the idea that care is needed in pregnancy is just as strange to them.[78]

Yet, the BHWC's annual report for the year 1936 recorded the interest of the middle-class Hindu women inhabiting the area around the Northern Centre in availing themselves of the antenatal services. It stated:

> It was very encouraging to find as the year proceeded how many middle class mothers availed themselves of the service of the antenatal clinic and brought their infants regularly to the welfare clinic for advice only. These mothers were sufficiently educated to follow the advice given and had the means to procure the kind of diets advised. Both they and the centre staff rejoiced in and appreciated the good results when the advice was followed ... The attendance at the antenatal clinic increased very much towards the end of the year and if this continues next year Northern Centre should show a high percentage of attendance for antenatal mothers.[79]

The report, however, focused on a small section of the middle-class women in a certain enclave in Calcutta and, hence, cannot be taken to represent the overwhelming response of the middle-class women to antenatal care.

The BHWC further observed that the centres based in areas dominated by Bengali Hindu population were more successful in antenatal work than those situated in Muslim-dominated areas. For instance, the *Shasthya Niketan* centre which was established in north Calcutta catered for a predominantly Hindu population of middle class and slum dwellers and, hence, recorded the highest percentage of antenatal attendance compared to other centres. Thus, religious character of the population constituted a powerful factor in determining the percentage of antenatal attendance in Calcutta in the 1930s. It was a fact further confirmed in 1931 by the Health Officer of the Corporation who ascribed the higher rates of infant mortality amongst the Muslims to a stricter practice of purdah that prevented Muslim women from seeking medical advice even when provided by female health visitors.[80]

The provision of antenatal care in the hospitals in Bengal was minimal in the period under review. As late as 1935, antenatal care at the Eden Hospital was stated to be far from satisfactory.[81] Yet the 1938–39 annual report of the CMC alluded to the 'popularity of our antenatal department'.[82] It was proudly stated that antenatal supervision of expectant mothers at the outpatients' department had lowered the rate of maternal morbidity and mortality including the percentage of puerperal sepsis. However, it was too radical a statement considering that even the antenatal clinic attached to the Lady Dufferin Victoria Hospital in Calcutta complained of having meagre success as only thirty patients on an average attended the clinic on a weekly basis and 'only one-tenth of cases admitted to Hospital had had any antenatal care'.[83] In the later years, however, antenatal care was prioritised by the Lady Dufferin Victoria Hospital to such an extent that antenatal cases were 'given the preference both for in-door and out-door treatment and no such case is ever refused'.[84]

Dr Sundari Mohan Das, a former councillor of the Calcutta Corporation, voiced the need for antenatal care in the hospitals. Das argued:

A Maternity Hospital does not mean a place for the delivery of labour cases only. We have to prepare the prospective mother for the strain of labour and giving birth to a healthy child. This means *Antenatal care*. But the care does not terminate with the termination of labour. We have to look after the mother and the child for a number of days to prevent childbirth complications and infantile mortality. This means *PostNatal Care*. All these mean expansion of the Hospital. At present, for want of accommodation, the ante and post-natal care have to suffer.[85]

By the 1940s, *Chittaranjan Seva Sadan* had developed an antenatal section at its Outpatient Department. It also boasted of an X-ray unit. However, the extent of use of X-ray technology for pelvic measurements or foetal monitoring during the period under study is hard to determine owing to paucity of documents.

The only significant hospital-based antenatal care was provided by the newly established *Sisumangal Pratisthan* (Childwelfare Institution) of the Ramakrishna Mission which was stated to have a 'system of smooth co-ordination of the activities of the institution in relation to the patients in general, viz., antenatal care, confinement (Home and hospital) and post-natal care'.[86] Sisumangal Pratisthan was also credited with possessing modern 'up-to-date appliances' for antenatal supervision and was said to have put 'great emphasis upon antenatal care, so much so that practically no care is undertaken without a proper course of ante-natal treatment'.[87] The institution also educated the expectant mothers through lectures, pamphlets and posters on diet, hygiene and infant care, as part of its antenatal work.[88] However, being a charitable institution, the success of the institution depended largely on the financial help received from the Calcutta Corporation and the 'support and sympathy' of the public.[89]

The trajectory of antenatal work in Bengal indicates that much of it remained outside the purview of doctors or obstetricians, although the need to bring pregnancy under medical supervision continued to be articulated by the medical professionals in the interwar years. Despite an increasing percentage of hospital births in the interwar years as alluded to in Chapter 3, hospital-based antenatal care was marginal, thereby suggesting lack of adequate infrastructure for such schemes and absence of public apathy towards the subject. Nevertheless, what started off as predominantly a municipal endeavour in the second decade of the twentieth century was pursued later by voluntary bodies such as the All India Institute of Hygiene and Public Health and the Bengal branch of the Red Cross Society in the 1930s. The Corporation's work being mainly confined to the slums and lower middle-class neighbourhoods of Calcutta, the intervention of the Red Cross Society implied a broadening of the social base of antenatal work. It incorporated the middle-class neighbourhoods in certain areas of the city. Yet, the scope of the antenatal work was circumscribed by the limited number of maternity and child welfare centres operating under the Bengal Health Welfare Committee.

## The constraints

Most of the districts outside Calcutta fell outside the purview of meaningful antenatal work executed by the municipalities and the voluntary bodies. This included the rural belts and the industrial areas. The nationalist press stressed the need for inclusion of antenatal and postnatal care schemes in the programmes of the Labour Welfare Organisation. It was proposed that antenatal work be carried out in dispensaries attached to every mill. Weekly examination of pregnant women in the mill areas was considered central to the clinic's work. Acquisition of basic instruments such as urine testing and blood pressure measuring apparatus, pelvimeter, speculum, scissors, dressing forceps was deemed indispensable to run the proposed antenatal clinic. It was insisted in the *Amrita Bazar Patrika* that 'as far as industrial areas are concerned, properly organised provision of antenatal and postnatal services for Mill labour does neither present any serious difficulty nor involve excessive outlay'.[90] Similarly, in the context of rural areas, it was argued that if the government provided a grant to the District Boards, then a 'rural Public Health Organisation' could be started which could initiate antenatal work in terms of home-visiting and providing mother-craft lessons to rural women.[91] Yet maternal mortality continued to figure as a potent national problem on the eve of independence and thereafter.

Antenatal work in Bengal remained fragmented even though its importance had been recognised across a wide spectrum of public debate on maternal and infant health from the 1920s. Despite the proliferation of maternity hospitals, admission of pregnant women before the onset of labour was rare and confined to a few hospitals. While assessing the failure of antenatal service to lower maternal mortality rates in Calcutta for the year 1936, the BHWC squarely placed the blame on the refusal of the expectant mother to follow the advice given by the antenatal clinics. However, according to Sundari Mohan Das, it was the inadequacy of financial resources rather than the lack of will of Bengali females to seek hospital treatment that hindered the expansion of maternity hospitals. The consequence was the failure of such hospitals to accommodate an increasing number of patients before the actual onset of labour.[92]

An enquiry in 1936 into the causes of maternal mortality in Calcutta conducted by Neal Edward, the professor of maternity and child welfare at the AIIHPH, revealed certain systemic weaknesses in the provision of antenatal care in Bengal. It revealed that the very few hospitals that conducted antenatal supervision lacked the provision of 'follow-up' in homes. The hospitals did not have enough beds for antenatal cases and also had no separate antenatal wards for the patients who were admitted to obstetric and other wards. Edward's study, therefore, concluded that the major hospitals and maternity homes admitted patients who were 'seen' for the first time during labour. In a similar vein, the quantity and quality of domiciliary antenatal work was also shown to be limited. In this connection, the study pointed out how antenatal supervision by maternity centres of patients who delivered at home was of a 'casual' nature. For those women who failed to show up or adhere to advices provided by the clinics, there was no systematic effort to bring them under supervision. Thus, it was concluded: 'The number of women in Calcutta at present who get systematic ante-natal care . . . is however limited to a few hundreds who come under the welfare centres and a certain number of others under the care of private practitioners.'[93]

The appointment of the Health Survey and Development Committee by the Government of India on 18 October 1943 under the chairmanship of Sir Joseph Bhore confirmed the deplorable rate of female mortality in India. It pointed out that 'on a conservative estimate, about 200,000 women died annually from causes arising out of childbirth in a year in British India. And that the number of those who suffered from varying degrees of disability resulting from the same causes must be many times that figure'.[94] It suggested uniformity in the supervision of pregnant women in the antenatal, natal and postnatal periods. It strongly recommended that the responsibility of the pregnant women in all the three stages of pregnancy be taken over by the same doctor, health visitor and midwife in each locality. It also stated that the appointment of more women doctors and health visitors would ensure the efficacy of the antenatal and postnatal schemes.

## Conclusion

The chapter analysed the major discursive strands around which the idea of antenatal care took shape in Bengal. Examining the writings on antenatal care in the Bengali popular print in the late nineteenth and early twentieth centuries, it demonstrated how the nineteenth-century Bengali writings, which were essentially non-medical in nature and constituted simple suggestions on care of pregnant women, were replaced in the twentieth century by more complex advices that subtly underscored the pathological nature of pregnancy and conveyed such notions in nationalist terms. The second major strand around which the idea of antenatal care crystallised in India was obstetric research on maternal morbidity and mortality that focused on the various diseases associated with pregnancy and insisted on the importance of antenatal care in detecting such diseases and eliminating them by timely and judicious medical intervention.

The chapter identified three factors responsible for the uneven nature of antenatal provision in Bengal: First, the cultural inhibitions of the average Bengali women debarred them from seeking antenatal consultation on a regular and sustained basis. Second, lack of financial resources or absence of aid from government impeded the expansion of the hospitals to include antenatal clinics. Third, the systematic implementation of antenatal care in Bengal was not hampered so much by the class divide as it was by a much stronger urban–rural divide.

The antenatal care provided by the municipalities and the voluntary organisations ensured accessibility of medical care during pregnancy to the poor and the lower middle class in the city. However, owing to the scant attention paid by the public health officials to the rural areas of Bengal, middle-class and poor women residing in the villages mostly remained deprived of the benefits of the modern health system till the end of the period of this study. Morbid portrayal of the sufferings of rural women under the grip of 'untrained', 'ignorant' and 'unscientific' dhais featured regularly in the nationalist press. Appeals for government intervention in training the dhais and co-opting them into modern health care system continued to be made.[95]

The half-hearted implementation of antenatal care schemes in late colonial Bengal does not, however, mean that there was an absence of public anxieties over maternal morbidity and mortality. The idea of science as the cornerstone of modern nation states accounts for the primacy accorded to the scientific management of birth in Bengal. Ideas on care of expectant mothers had been in vogue in Bengali popular print media in the nineteenth century and were standardised further in the twentieth century. Furthermore, research on antenatal care and the specificities of tropical diseases related to childbirth, and the emphasis on pelvimetry and urine tests enabled the emergence of new perceptions on the management of pregnancy and childbirth. Female body formed the nuclei around which a medical discourse was forged that defined the 'national' problems of maternal and infant mortality from a global perspective. Yet the actual care of pregnant women remained in the hands of health visitors and voluntary workers who were insufficiently qualified and trained to address the needs of the Bengali female population on a sustained basis. Childbirth was not completely medicalised in India till the 1980s.[96] Yet as the chapter argues, a beginning had been made in the early twentieth century, at least in discourse, if not entirely in practice.

## Notes

1 R.W. Johnstone, 'Fifty Years of Midwifery', *The British Medical Journal*, Vol.1, No.4644, 1950, 12.
2 Ibid.
3 Ann Oakley, *The Captured Womb: A History of the Medical Care of Pregnant Women*, Oxford and New York: Basil Blackwell, 1984, 25.
4 J.W. Ballantyne, 'An Address on the New Midwifery: Preventive and Reparative Obstetrics', *The British Medical Journal*, Vol.1, No.3250, 1923, 617–621.
5 Johnstone, 'Fifty Years', 13.

6  Ibid.
7  W.R. Arney, *Power and the Profession of Obstetrics*, Chicago and London: Chicago University Press, 1982, 100. Also see Elaine Papps and Mark Olsen, *Doctoring Childbirth and Regulating Midwifery in New Zealand: A Foucaldian Perspective*, Palmerstone North: Dunmore Press, 1997.
8  Arney, *Power and the Profession of Obstetrics*, 8.
9  Arthur S. Macnalty, 'Britain's Development of Preventive Medicine', *Canadian Journal of Public Health*, Vol.35, No.1, January 1944, 10–15.
10  G.F. McCleary, *The Maternity and Child Welfare Movement*, London: P.S. King & Son Ltd, 1935, 50.
11  Johnstone, 'Fifty Years', 13.
12  Oakley, *Captured Womb*.
13  Oakley, *Captured Womb*, 12.
14  '*Dhatribidya: Garbhabasthyay Prasutir Susrusa* (Midwifery: Care of Pregnant Women)', *Bamabodhini Patrika*, Vol.3, No.51, November 1867, 616–619.
15  '*Grihasiksha: Matrigarbha* (Home Education: The Womb of a Pregnant Woman)', *Paricarika*, Vol.14, No.11, February 1892, 252–254.
16  Haranath Ray, *Dhatri-Siksha Samgraha* (Midwife's Vade-Mecum), Calcutta: Bengal Law Report Press, 1887.
17  Dr Kartik Chandra Basu, '*Suchana* (Beginning)', *Svasthya Samacara*, Vol. 1, No.1, April–May 1912, 3–4.
18  David Arnold, *Colonising the Body: State Medicine and Epidemic Disease in Nineteenth-Century India*, Berkeley, Los Angeles and London: University of California Press, 1993, 294.
19  Amand Routh, 'Observations on the Toxaemias of Pregnancy, and on Eugenics from the Obstetrics Standpoint', *The British Medical Journal*, Vol.2, No.2740, July 1913, 17–20.
20  'Some Economic Aspects of Ante-natal Pathology', *The British Medical Journal*, Vol.1, No.2060, June 1900, 1547–1548.
21  Routh, 'Observations on the Toxaemias of Pregnancy'.
22  Editorial, 'Mother and Child – Their Health', *The Calcutta Medical Journal*, Vol.9, 1915, 79–81.
23  '*Garbhinir Kartabya* (Duties of a Pregnant Woman)', *Svasthya Samacara*, Vol.5, No.12, 1916, 333–340.
24  For instance see '*Garbhabasthyay Satarkata* (Caution During Pregnancy)', *Svasthya Samacara*, Vol.9, No.9, December 1920, 204–207.
25  Dr Frederick Truby King was a New Zealand-based health reformer and the founder of the Plunket Society (1907) for the promotion of health of women and children. King made antenatal care in New Zealand 'fashionable' by persuading women of 'high society' to attend maternity clinics. See Lawrence D. Longo and Christina M. Thomsen, 'Prenatal Care and Its Evolution in America', in Philip K. Wilson, ed. *Childbirth: The Medicalisation of Obstetrics: Personnel, Practice and Instruments*, New York and London: Garland Publishing House, 1996, 168. Francis James Browne (1879–1968) was an Irish obstetrician who worked with Ballantyne in Edinburgh in the post-1918 years, served as the first professor of obstetrics in the University College Hospital, London and later moved to Sydney. Browne's interest chiefly lay in antenatal and postnatal care on which he wrote extensively till his death. Browne's books on antenatal care were

widely read by medical students and were used in the works of Bengali doctors trained in the United Kingdom and other European countries.

26 Girindra Krishna Mitra, *Prasuti o Santan*, Calcutta: Bengal Publishing Home, 1929, Introduction.

27 See, for instance, Poonam Bala, ' "Nationalising Medicine": The Changing Paradigm of Ayurveda in British India', in Poonam Bala, ed. *Contesting Colonial Authority: Medicine and Indigenous Responses in Nineteenth and Twentieth Century India*, Maryland: Lexington Books, 2012.

28 Mitra, *Prasuti o Santan*.

29 For instance, *Bangalakshmi* published articles on antenatal care in the 1920s. See for instance, Miss Hansa, '*Garbhinir Gyatabya* (Things a Pregnant Woman Should Know)', *Bangalakshmi*, Vol.2, No.4, 1926, 130–132.

30 V.B. Green-Armytage, 'Ante-Natal Care', *The Indian Medical Gazette*, Vol.59, August 1924, 415.

31 Green-Armytage, 'Ante-Natal Care'.

32 V.B. Green-Armytage, *Tropical Midwifery: Labour Room Clinics*, Calcutta and Simla: Thacker, Spink & Co, 1928.

33 Green-Armytage, *Tropical Midwifery*, 1.

34 Subodh Mitra, 'Ante-Natal Care', *Amrita Bazar Patrika*, 13 April 1941.

35 Ibid.

36 A.C. Chatterjee, 'Mother and the Child', *Amrita Bazar Patrika*, 13 April 1941.

37 Gorachand Nandi, 'Antenatal Care', *Calcutta Medical Review*, Vol.4, No.4, 1941, 121–132.

38 Mitra, 'Ante-Natal Care'. Also see Alison M. Headwards, 'Care of Expectant Mothers', *Amrita Bazar Patrika*, 13 April 1941.

39 Oakley, *Captured Womb*, 63.

40 M.I. Balfour, 'A Comment on the Report on Maternal Mortality During Childbirth in England by Dr Janet Campbell of the Ministry of Health, with a Reference to Maternal Mortality in India', *The Indian Medical Gazette*, Vol.59, December 1924, 621–624. The report does not mention the sex of the doctor. It can however be assumed that she was referring to both the male and female medical professionals.

41 The Indian Research Fund Association was established in 1911 as a body promoting medical research in India and remained the principal body conducting medical research till independence. After independence; it was renamed as the Indian Council for Medical Research. For details, see Ward Morehouse, *Science in India*, Bombay: Administrative Staff College of India, 1971.

42 *Maternal Mortality in Childbirth in India: A Summary of the Investigations Conducted Under the Indian Research Fund Association, 1925*, Calcutta: Government of India Central Publication Branch, 1928.

43 'Maternal Mortality in Childbirth in India', 1.

44 'Maternal Mortality in Childbirth in India', 12.

45 'F.E.A.T.M Congress: Obstetrics and Gynaecology', *Indian Medical Gazette*, Vol.63, April 1928, 216.

46 *Annual Report of the All India Institute of Hygiene and Public Health (AIIHPH)*, 1938, Calcutta: Government of India Press, 1939, 48–49.

47 A.M. Mallick, 'The Pelvis in the Female and Its Progressive Development (as Studied from Some Indian Cases)', *The Calcutta Medical Journal*,

Vol.9, 1915, 41–54. Also Chapter 2 has shown Kedarnath Das's research on pelvis of Bengali women which led him to modify the Simpson forceps and design the famous 'Bengal forceps' for Bengali females. For details, see Chapter 2.

48 Grace Stapleton, 'Pelvic Measurements in Indian Women', *The Indian Medical Gazette*, Vol.60, December 1925, 560–561. Subsequently published in *Journal of the Association of Medical Women in India*, Vol.15, No.2, 1927, 8–11.

49 Kathleen Vaughan, 'The Shape of the Pelvic Brim as a Determining Factor in Childbirth', *The British Medical Journal*, Vol.2, No.3698, 1931, 939–941.

50 Hemangini Sen, '*Svasthya Samasya* (Health Problems)', *Bangalakshmi*, Vol.3, No.7, 1929, 533–535.

51 Maneesha Lal, 'Purdah as Pathology: Gender and Circulation of Medical Knowledge in Colonial India', in Sarah Hodges, ed. *Reproductive Health in India: History, Politics, Controversies*, Delhi: Orient Longman, 2006.

52 Lal, 'Purdah as Pathology', 87.

53 Oakley, *Captured Womb*, 79.

54 Ranajit Sinha, 'Some Preventive Aspects of Obstetrics', *Journal of the Indian Medical Association*, Vol.10, No.7, 1941. Also see, '*Prasuti Hatya* (Death of Pregnant Woman)', *Byabosa O Banijya*, Vol.14, No.9, 1934, 718–719.

55 'Maternity and Child Welfare Work in India', *Journal of the Indian Medical Association*, Vol.8, No.1, October 1938, 38–39.

56 Margaret Balfour and Shakuntala Talpade, 'The Influence of Diet on Pregnancy and Early Infant Mortality in India', *The Indian Medical Gazette*, Vol.LXVII, No.1, 1932, 601–606. Also, Rao Sahib, 'Deficiency Diseases and Pregnancy', *Indian Medical Record*, March 1944, 65–70.

57 'Clinical and Scientific Proceedings: Calcutta Branch, Pregnancy Anaemia in India', *The British Medical Journal*, Vol.1, No.3726, 1932, 1031–1032.

58 G.G. Jolly, 'The Need for Co-operation in the Medical Health Services of India with Special Reference to Maternity and Child Welfare', *The Indian Medical Gazette*, April 1940, 237.

59 'Editorials: Medical Profession and Maternal and Child Welfare Work', *Calcutta Medical Journal*, Vol.41, No.6, 1944, 196–199.

60 H.M. Crake, *Report of the Health Officer of Calcutta*, Calcutta: The Corporation Press, 1913.

61 Crake, *Report of the Health Officer of Calcutta*, 1914.

62 Crake, *Report of the Health Officer of Calcutta*, 1916.

63 Crake, *Report of the Health Officer of Calcutta*, 1920, 1921 and 1922.

64 Crake, *Report of the Health Officer of Calcutta*, 1922.

65 'Calcutta Milk Supply', *The Amrita Bazar Patrika*, 28 September 1908.

66 'All India Cow Conference', *The Amrita Bazar Patrika*, 31 December 1920; 'Preservation of our Cattle Wealth', *The Amrita Bazar Patrika*, 31 December 1920.

67 Brojendranath Ganguly, 'Dugdha Samasya', *Sachitra Sisir*, Vol.2, No. 16, 1924, 544–545.

68 Ibid.

69 Crake, *Report of the Health Officer of Calcutta*, 1914, 23.
70 Luise Gompertz, 'In a Calcutta Slum: Taking Care of Mother and Child', *The Calcutta Municipal Gazette*, The Twelfth Health Number, 26 April 1941, 61–70.
71 *Bengal Public Health Report, 1936*, Alipore, Bengal: Bengal Government Press, 1938, 101–102.
72 '*Mahila Samitir Sangbad* (News from Women's Organization)', *Bangalakshmi*, Vol.3, No.2, 1927. 'Lecture by Suprava Mukherjie', *Bangalakshmi*, Vol.3, No.2, 1927.
73 *Annual Report, AIIHPH*, 1936.
74 *Annual Report, AIIHPH*, 1938.
75 *Bengal Health Welfare Committee*, Annual Report, Indian Red Cross Society, 1936, 4.
76 S.B. Ray, 'Maternity and Child Welfare: Neglect in India, a Scheme for Calcutta Industrial Areas', *Amrita Bazar Patrika*, 11 December 1939.
77 *Bengal Health Welfare Committee*, 9.
78 Ruth Young, *Ante Natal Work in India: A Handbook for Nurses, Midwives and Health Visitors*, Maternity and Child Welfare Bureau: Indian Red Cross Society, 1931, 1.
79 *Bengal Health Welfare Committee*, 12.
80 T.N. Majumdar, *Report of the Health Officer of Calcutta*, Calcutta: The Corporation Press, 1931, 8.
81 *The Centenary of the Medical College Bengal*, Medical College Centenary Volume Sub-Committee, 1935, Chapter 4, 98.
82 *Annual Report on the Working of the Medical College, Calcutta, 1938–39*, Alipore: Bengal Government Press, 1939.
83 *Annual Report of the National Association for Supplying Medical Aid by Women to the Women of India*, 1936, Simla: Government of India Press, 1937, 67.
84 *Annual Report of the National Association for Supplying Medical Aid by Women to the Women of India*, 1940, 88.
85 Sundari Mohan Das, 'A Plea for Calcutta Hospitals', *The Calcutta Municipal Gazette*, 15th Anniversary Number, 16 December 1939, 16.
86 Birendranath De, 'Maternity Work and the Shishumangal Prathisthan', *Prabuddha Bharata*, Vol.LXVII, No.1, January 1942, 45–50.
87 Ibid.
88 *Ramakrishna Mission: Sisumangal Pratishthan: A Maternity Hospital and Child Welfare Centre*, Report for the Year 1939, Calcutta: Secretary Ramakrishna Mission Sisumangal Pratishthan, 1940, 13.
89 Ibid., 9.
90 Ray, 'Maternity and Child Welfare'.
91 J.N. Chakraborty, 'Fight Against Infant Mortality', *Amrita Bazar Patrika*, 25 September 1937.
92 Das, 'A Plea for Calcutta Hospitals'.
93 M.I. Neal Edwards, *Report of an Enquiry into the Causes of Maternal Mortality in Calcutta*, Health Bulletin No.27, Delhi: Manager of Publications, 1956.
94 *Report of the Health Survey and Development Committee*, Delhi: Government of India Publications Department, January 1946, Chapter 8, 97.

95 See, for instance, J.N. Chakraborty, 'Fight Against Infant Mortality' and 'Bengal Maternity Services: Deplorable State', *Amrita Bazar Patrika*, 17 April 1941.
96 Imrana Qadeer, 'Continuities and Discontinuities in Public Health: The Indian Experience', in Amiya Kumar Bagchi and Krishna Soman, eds. *Maladies, Preventives, and Curatives: Debates in Public Health in India*, New Delhi: Tulika Books, 2005.

# Conclusion

The history of the medicalisation of childbirth in colonial Bengal is embedded in a complex process of modernisation that traversed two major phases in the social history of Bengal: the reformist phase in the late nineteenth century and the nationalist phase in the twentieth century. The book has drawn explicit parallels between the evolution of a professional middle class in Bengal and their access to western education and the concomitant rise of a medical culture spurred by the foundation of the Calcutta Medical College (CMC). The history of medicalisation of childbirth is located at the crucial conjuncture of the two emerging discourses: a discourse on modernity that inspired and in certain instances forced a reconsideration of existing sociocultural categories. Second, a new medical discourse that caused existing parameters of health practices to change or modify in keeping with the new medical culture. While modernity as an embodiment of rationalist scientific thought was the key ideological driver of change through the reformist and the nationalist phase, the mode of expression had significantly changed. In charting the transition of midwifery from a female-centred event to a medical one, the book has explored three discursive strands: (1) it has located the urge for modernising birthing practices within the transforming sociocultural milieu of nineteenth-century Bengal that was steered solely by the self-improving drive of the western-educated bhadralok; (2) it has traced the various axes around which midwifery education was instituted and sustained in Bengal; (3) it has delineated the contours of professionalisation of obstetrics and the political imperatives shaping it.

The reformist initiatives to improve childbearing practices in the second half of the nineteenth century were essentially driven by a modernist middle-class consciousness. The centrality of the rhetoric of science and rationality in shaping this modernist middle-class identity emerged as the pivotal factor engineering a series of socio-economic transformations in Bengal. The reconfiguration of domesticity and conjugality was part of this transformative process. Such reform initiatives also emerged as part of self-improving drive of the middle class who sought to challenge and negate the colonial insinuations that Bengali customs were decadent and barbaric. Improvement of birthing practices became an integral part of such reform agendas. The foundation of the CMC and the medical culture it fostered acted as powerful catalysts in further stoking the curiosity of the middle-class Bengalis and inspiring them to interrogate the existing health practices.

The print culture played a central role in creating extremely fluid and autonomous spaces for the middle class to question pre-existing practices and articulate new ideas. The book has linked popular reading culture to the modernisation of birthing practices to show how the ideas debated and negotiated in print impinged on the psyche of the readers that included a significant section of literate female readers from the late nineteenth century. The loss of infant life that was beginning to be recognised as a matter of concern by the Bengali males from the second half of the nineteenth century was attributed to the ignorant practices of the uneducated Bengali women and the dhais. As female education was gaining ground in Bengal, the bhadralok utilised this opportune moment and deployed the power of print to teach western scientific principles of midwifery to the middle-class women as part of educating and enlightening them as mothers.

The earliest essays on scientific midwifery that were being disseminated through the pages of women's magazines constituted the first major attempt at redefining birth as a medical phenomenon. By hinting at the pathological underpinnings of the birthing process, the central message that emerged through the writings was: pregnancy and childbirth were something more than the dhais alone could comprehend and manage. Under the impact of the new clinical discourse introduced by western medical science taught at CMC, such writings boldly questioned the validity of existing birthing practices derided as irrational and unscientific. The definition of pregnancy as a pathological process, once again, acquired primacy in the nationalist discourse on maternal and infant welfare in the twentieth century.

The second major discursive strand of the book revolved around the process through which midwifery was constituted into a medical discourse and subsequently institutionalised in Bengal in the late nineteenth and early twentieth centuries. The book has demonstrated how the delayed response of Bengal in introducing and improving the standards of midwifery education as compared to Madras was, to a substantial extent, due to the disproportionate importance attached to the Indian custom of seclusion in justifying the initial reluctance of the CMC authorities to allocate funds for a separate midwifery class. Seclusion was a convenient trope used by the government in prioritising the teaching of dhais at the cost of ignoring the male students despite all their readiness to learn midwifery. Later, the same logic of seclusion was deployed by few liberal British administrative officials and a section of the Brahmo reformers to argue in favour of admitting female physicians to the Medical College.

The book has addressed a major historical void that stemmed from the contention that women doctors were the sole agents in the medicalisation of childbirth owing to their easy accessibility to the Indian zenanas. While women doctors played a major role in providing medical aid to women in zenanas, male doctors' contribution was no less significant. As professors of midwifery, researchers, composers of tracts on the science of reproduction and nationalists seeking to initiate a public debate in support of modern maternity care in the interest of the nation, the role of the male doctors remained more ideological though less directly participatory in the realm of actual medical practice. By publishing easily readable monographs and scientific tracts on midwifery in Bengali language that were meant for the instruction of dhais and ordinary middle-class readers or by experimenting with surgical techniques on female patients in hospitals, the male doctors consolidated the theoretical and scientific foundations of the newly evolved science of obstetrics. Cloaking their arguments in nationalist rhetoric, they advocated cautious use of forceps in obstructed labour, defended caesarean sections and spoke in favour of antenatal care for preventing maternal and infant mortality. Emerged as nationalists in the 1920s, they defended and overhauled the structure of midwifery education in the medical colleges against charges of inadequacy and defective training made by the General Medical Council of England.

Examining the ideological context in which obstetrics was constituted into a profession constituted the third discursive strand of the book. The spotlight has particularly been on the role of medical professionals who framed a public discourse on maternal and child welfare by drawing upon the rhetoric of motherhood and global eugenic notions on the centrality of race in national regeneration. In the years following the First World War, concerns for maternal and infant health that acquired national importance in England impinged upon the nationalist sensibilities of the Bengali middle class. Consequently, motherhood was drawn into the centre of an emotionally charged nationalist discourse.

The emergence of secular politics from the 1920s and the pressure from international bodies such as the League of Nations further sharpened the nationalist focus on infant and maternal welfare as the key to national efficiency while at the same time creating a conducive environment for the penetration of international ideas on health into the national milieu. The dynamic interface between the national and the global featured recurrently in the writings of medical men. Examples from western countries abound in such writings. Yet in absorbing global ideas, the medical professionals and the middle-class bhadralok sought to conceal the western origin of such ideas and project them as part of indigenous medical tradition.

In delineating the contours of the process by which the profession of obstetrics was constituted in Bengal, the study has drifted away from conventional narratives pivoting around the institutionalisation of Dufferin Fund and instead looked closely at the role of the local government. The novelty of the midwifery schemes introduced by the Calcutta Municipal Corporation drew the lower-middle-class women within the fold of standardised professional maternal care. In forging coordination between public health officials (chiefly the health visitors) and the medical professionals the Corporation enabled the consolidation of medical/professional control over the process of pregnancy. The schemes such as home-visits to pregnant women's houses by health visitors or instituting domiciliary midwifery services to ensure professional attendance at birth were remarkable measures, the first of their kind that quickly soared in popularity. The participation of indigenous medical men and nationalist leaders in formulating midwifery schemes ensured provision of western allopathic medical aid to the lower-middle-class women as the only viable way to curtail maternal and infant mortality in Bengal.

Concerns over maternal and infant mortality led to the promotion of the idea of antenatal care in Bengali popular print, particularly in the writings of the Bengali doctors contributing to health journals and women's magazines. While rudimentary ideas of antenatal care were already in vogue from the late nineteenth century as evident from the sporadic publication of essays entitled *Garbhinir Paricharya* ('Care of Pregnant Women'), in the interwar years, such writings in the press, popular journals and lectures delivered at the baby shows and health welfare exhibitions acquired technological undertones. Birth was explicitly defined as a pathological condition that required medical supervision and professional attendance. Diseases associated with pregnancy were highlighted in research on maternal mortality that were simultaneously backed by claims of the medical professionals that diseases in pregnancy could be eradicated antenatally.

Yet there were important limitations that throttled the process of medicalisation of childbirth in colonial Bengal. The book has demonstrated that antenatal care in Bengal in the 1940s had less to do with technological dominance and more with prenatal advice about diet and hygiene by health visitors during home-visits. Hospital-based antenatal care was extremely limited that accounted for the preponderance of the Calcutta Municipal Corporation and voluntary bodies such as the Bengal branch of the Indian Red Cross Society in delivering antenatal care in the 1940s. Pelvimetry, urine test and inspection of female body were not yet introduced on a regular basis, such tests being only available at a few institutions such as the Ramakrishna Sisumangal Pratisthan and the antenatal clinics established under the auspices of the Bengal branch of the Indian Red Cross Society. The inadequacy of financial resources, systemic weaknesses in the hospital-based antenatal care and, lastly, the lack of awareness of women of the value of antenatal care constituted major constraints in limiting the scope of antenatal supervision in Bengal.

Many of the endeavours made by medical professionals, voluntary bodies, public health authorities and the municipal corporation relied heavily on public subscription and, hence, remained susceptible to financial constraints throughout the period under consideration. Maternal and child welfare continued to be brushed aside as relatively insignificant as late as the 1930s. The government officials explained this lack of interest by citing prevalent social prejudices including the cultural practice of seclusion that, according to them, rendered any state-sponsored initiative futile. But that argument certainly did not explain the state's apathy at a juncture when Bengali society was displaying greater 'hospital-mindedness' and willingness to embrace western form of maternal care.

In conclusion therefore, the study identified three trends in the professionalisation of obstetrics in Bengal in the nationalist period that continued unabated in the post-colonial period: First, the rising popularity of the hospital deliveries in the interwar years that could partly be ascribed to a growing number of maternity homes and hospitals in urban areas during this phase. The overarching factor was, however, the growing middle-class faith in allopathic medical system that was associated with modernity. Second, the contribution of the male and female doctors towards expanding the sphere of professionalised obstetrics. In promoting research and proposing remedies to curtail maternal morbidity and mortality, the female doctors did not deviate majorly from male-dominated medical perspectives and practices. Hence, the professional space that emerged in the interwar years was more of a shared one than being stringently demarcated along gender lines. Nationalist and eugenic concerns for loss of infant and maternal life led the middle-class elites, nationalist leaders, Indian feminists and the medical profession to argue in favour of medical supervision over pregnancy and childbirth. Third, the existence of a wide urban–rural divide was a major barrier impeding the accessibility of modern health care services to all. It can hardly be denied that maternal care in urban Bengal was being modernised and incorporated into western allopathic medical structure by the end of colonial rule. Western allopathic medical practice significantly touched upon the lives of the middle-class women who, from the early part of the twentieth century, were beginning to recognise the worth of scientific management of birth. In the interwar years, it drew the lower-middle-class women including slum dwellers, not strictly bound by the rules of purdah, into its fold. Yet modern maternity care remained confined to urban Bengal while rural areas remained largely outside the pale of institutionalised midwifery services.

# Afterword

The government's apathy towards maternal health was part of its indifference towards public health in general, a trend that continued into the post-colonial period. Despite the centrality of public health issues in the National Planning Committee formed by the Indian National Congress in 1938 to outline the contours of an independent India, the health of the population, as Sunil Amrith has argued, was merely an instrument for the post-colonial government to promote its higher aim of creating a planned industrialised state. It was, thus, a 'story of the instruments becoming an end in themselves and trumping the fundamental idioms, or values, of health'.[1] Contrary to the recommendations of the Bhore Committee that rural India be made the focus of the post-colonial health structure, what emerged instead was a 'doctor-based, urban-biased' health care system.[2]

In the arena of women's reproductive health, although maternal and child health care services were integrated by the Government of India into the First Five Year (1951–56) and Second Five Year (1956–61) plans, the spotlight shifted chiefly onto birth control and eugenics. It was argued that frequent pregnancies caused strain on the health of the mother leading to maternal and infant deaths and the birth of weak children. The key to safeguard maternal health, therefore, lay in controlling pregnancy by contraceptive methods. Increasing demand was made for including birth control in maternal and child health services.[3] While birth control had been the subject of fervent public discourse in the early part of the twentieth century it was promoted chiefly through elitist endeavours and mediation of international agencies and western social activists such as Marie Stopes, Margaret Sanger, Edith How-Martyn and Eileen Palmer. Towards the end of colonial rule, birth control was integrated into the National Planning Committee's efforts in the creation of a healthy race that would contribute towards national efficiency and development. Thus, birth control emerged as a key official policy of the post-colonial government. Population control through state intervention and deployment of modern reproductive technologies was endorsed by the First Five Year Plan in 1951 and received enthusiastic support from western aid agencies such as the Rockefeller Foundation, Ford Foundation and USAID.

However, birth control became the focal point of active state policy only from the Third Five Year Plan in 1961 and was administered under a separate department of Family Planning created in 1966. As Mohan Rao argues, family planning was allotted a budget of Rs 0.5 billion in the Third Five Year Plan as against a modest Rs 6.5 million in the First Five Year Plan, denoting its centrality in the health administration in post-colonial India at the expense of marginalising other vital areas of public health.[4] Maternal and child health was eventually integrated into family planning services during the Fifth Five Year Plan (1974–79) with the objective of providing minimum public services to pregnant women, lactating mothers and pre-school children. Yet as Rao argues, the entire public health infrastructure, in the post-colonial years, was dominated by concerns for population control and family planning measures. The consequence was the spawning of a private sector in health that, according to Rao, was largely 'exploitative' and 'unregulated'.[5]

What then was the status of medicalisation of childbirth in post-colonial Bengal? A brief review of the post-colonial maternal health services in West Bengal reveals a continuity of trend that confirms the findings of this study. A health survey conducted in West Bengal in 1955 by the Indian Statistical Institute revealed a 'very unsatisfactory' picture of the maternal health care services in Bengal. Despite claiming to be 'exploratory' in nature rather than being 'very reliable', the report nonetheless revealed that about 24 per cent of the rural deliveries and 20 per cent of the urban ones took place in Bengal without professional attendance of any sort, whereas those attended by dhais constituted 76 per cent of the rural deliveries and 25 per cent of the urban ones.[6] In the 1960s, however, West Bengal was much ahead of other states in India in terms of hospital deliveries in urban areas.[7]

Moni Nag's comparative study of West Bengal and Kerala in the 1950s and 1960s is more revealing. Nag's research based on the data collected for the years 1959 and 1964 reveal that rural Bengal lagged behind Kerala in terms of utilisation of preventive and curative medical health care facilities including maternal and health services. Nag has explained this difference in terms of the differing literacy levels of the two states and degree of the political awareness of the rural poor in demanding improved medical facilities. Bengal despite being ahead

of most states in India in the sphere of higher education has historically harboured an urban-elitist bias that accounts for the neglect of
primary education in the rural areas. Moreover, lower female literacy
rates amongst the rural Bengali females also explain their diffidence in
seeking maternal and child health services. This was in sharp contrast
to Kerala which has the highest literacy rate in India.[8] In terms of
statistics also, the rural–urban divide in Bengal appears all the more
glaring when compared to Kerala. For instance, the National Sample
Survey[9] data shows that for the years 1964–65, while the percentage
of rural women attended by physicians or qualified nurses in Kerala
was 16 per cent, it was only 3 per cent in West Bengal. By contrast, in
the urban areas, where the percentage of urban women attended by
skilled professionals was 35 per cent in Kerala, it was 42 per cent in
West Bengal. Similarly, while the percentage of institutionalised (hospital) birth was 13 per cent in rural Kerala, it was a low 6 per cent in
rural Bengal. In the urban areas, by sharp contrast, Bengal recorded
50 per cent institutionalised delivery whereas Kerala recorded only
32 per cent. Thus, childbirth in Bengal remains more medicalised in
the urban areas than in rural parts.

The most significant theme in the story of childbirth in post-colonial
Bengal is therefore the urban middle class penchant for institutional
delivery and modern maternal care. Henrike Donner's ethnographic
enquiry into the middle-class birthing patterns in post-colonial Calcutta shows that by the 1960s, middle-class families in Calcutta had
largely accepted medical intervention in childbirth as safe. The mush-
rooming of a large number of private nursing homes in the 1960s, that
ensured a more intimate doctor–patient relationship and less 'anonymity' than state-run hospitals, drew more middle-class women towards
the medicalised model of childbirth.[10] It falls in line with the central
argument of this study about the hegemonic grip of western-style midwifery on middle-class consciousness. By the 1980s, birth in private
nursing homes evolved into a status symbol for the middle class in
Calcutta, a trend accentuated by the privatisation of medical care in
the 1980s and 1990s. In the context of these major structural transformations, Donner has noted two major shifts in the birthing patterns of
the Bengali middle class in the 1990s. The first was the shift in the site
of birth from home to private nursing homes in a manner that established the 'supremacy of medicalised model of birth' so that 'deliveries
and medical care for pregnant women became a matter of prestige for
her affines'. The second shift was the rising preponderance of the interventionist obstetrics to the extent that it established caesarean section
as the preferred form of delivery for middle-class women.[11] Donner

has explained the growing preference for caesarean section not only in terms of the broader structural changes but also very much in terms of the personal choice and agency of women that were intricately shaped by class and 'intra-household relations'.[12] Donner's findings fall in line with Brigitte Jordan's argument that the

> unquestioned superior status of biomedicine leads to a principled, rather than reasoned, devaluation of indigenous obstetric procedures and practitioners. Biomedicine in many developing countries has acquired a symbolic value that is independent of its use value. It has come to symbolise modernisation and progress.[13]

Given Bengal's deep-rooted association with colonial modernity and western education, it is not hard to comprehend the reason behind the middle class's inclination towards hospital deliveries.

A more recent and comprehensive picture of the status of medicalised model of birth in post-colonial Bengal is provided by the findings of an extensive research conducted by the National Family Health Survey and the Reproductive and Child Health Programme in the 1990s. It reveals that in the 1990s, almost 60 per cent of deliveries took place in homes, while 40 per cent took place in hospitals. Bengal had a greater percentage of rural women reporting 'normal' delivery than urban women to the extent that the rate of normal birth sharply plummeted in the urban areas. It was estimated that only 833 of every 1,000 urban mothers were reported to have 'normal' delivery against a national average of 891. More interestingly, operative interventions during delivery were found to be more frequent in urban areas than in rural areas. Thus, it was calculated that only 13 out of 1,000 rural women in West Bengal reported operation during delivery against a national average of 23. In sharp contrast, the overall trend of operative intervention during delivery was much higher in West Bengal than the national average. While 133 out of every 1,000 urban mothers underwent operation during delivery, the national average was only 76.[14] In the sphere of antenatal care, while 75.3 per cent of the Bengali pregnant women received at least one antenatal check-up which was considered better than all India average, only 19 per cent of pregnant women went through a comprehensive antenatal care programme. In this respect, West Bengal was behind nine of the fifteen major states in India.[15]

Given the dominance of hospital births in urban Bengal, it is no wonder that the feminist health movement that evolved in India in the 1980s, despite drawing succour from similar movements in the West, significantly diverged from the latter, the most crucial point of divergence being the palpable absence of any demand for home-birth or natural childbirth movement. In the West, the central objective of the women's health movement that evolved in the 1970s has been to wrest the control of birth management from the highly technologised, male-controlled medical establishment and restore it to women. Feminist assertion of women's fundamental right to be in control of their body and reproduction was the salient feature of the home-birth movement that developed in America and other western countries. The health movement in India, on the other hand, crystallised around opposing invasive reproductive technologies that allegedly tampered with women's reproductive functions. The key issues were curbing unethical clinical trials of contraceptives, putting bans on hazardous drugs that could be used as abortifacients and, most significantly, campaigning against medical procedures like amniocentesis that could be deployed for sex determination and female infanticide.[16]

From the 1990s, however, scholars have questioned the sagacity of 'superficial' medical interventions in problems related to reproductive health that have deeper social and economic roots and, hence, lie beyond 'conventional medical boundaries'. In the absence of genuine State initiatives to understand the epidemiological basis of reproductive health problems or to analyse the impact of major industrial and agricultural policy shifts on the health of women, medical interventions in most cases would prove to be unwarranted and extremely unproductive.[17] Such scholarly concerns have largely gone unheeded in policy-formulation pertaining to health in India. However, certain non-governmental organisations, in recent years, have directed their efforts towards promoting the knowledge of the indigenous dhais without directly challenging the dominant biomedical paradigm. They have been relentlessly working towards integrating the dhais in a more inclusive health care system that will be premised on the co-existence of the indigenous and the western framework of knowledge rather than the latter dominating and redefining the parameters of the former. However, such efforts are more visible in Gujarat, Tamil Nadu, Jharkhand and Maharashtra than in Bengal.[18]

The study has shown the extreme polarisation in colonial Bengal along urban rural lines that hampered the spread of modern maternity care amongst the masses. That trend has continued into the postcolonial period as well. While a section of the Bengali population represented by the educated middle class prefer and enjoy privileged access to technologised medical care and all that is less painful and more convenient, the bulk of the population residing in the country-side remain outside the ambit of even the most elementary form of maternal services. Perhaps herein lay the greatest failure of national-ism, the failure to integrate the vast mass of people whom the nation claimed to represent. As Partha Chatterjee has aptly argued:

> The formation of a hegemonic 'national culture' was necessarily built upon a system of exclusions. Ideas of freedom, equality and cultural refinement went hand in hand with a set of dichotomies which systematically excluded from the new life of the nation the vast masses of people whom the dominant elite would represent and lead, but who would never be culturally integrated with their leaders.[19]

## Notes

1 Sunil Amrith, 'Political Culture of Health in India: A Historical Perspec-tive', *Economic and Political Weekly*, Vol.42, No.2, 2007, 119.
2 Mohan Rao, *From Population Control to Reproductive Health: Malthu-sian Arithmetic*, New Delhi: Sage Publications, 2004, 25.
3 Ibid., 19–20.
4 Ibid., 32.
5 Ibid., 15.
6 S.J. Poti, M.V. Raman, S. Biswas and B. Chakraborty, 'A Pilot Health Survey in West Bengal:1955', *Sankhya, The Indian Journal of Statistics*, Vol.21, No.1/2, 1959, 146.
7 Moni Nag, 'Impact of Social and Economic Development on Mortality: Comparative Study of Kerala and West Bengal', *Economic and Political Weekly*, Vol.18, Nos.19–21, 1983, 877–900.
8 Ibid.
9 National Sample Survey was the only organisation in India after independ-ence that collected socio-economic statistics on a national scale.
10 Henrike Donner, *Domestic Goddesses: Maternity, Globalisation and Middle-Class Identity in Contemporary India*, London: Ashgate, 2008, 104.
11 Ibid., 117.
12 Ibid., 115.
13 Brigitte Jordan, 'Technology Transfer in Obstetrics: Theory and Practice in Developing Countries', Michigan State University, Working Paper 126, September 1986, 2.
14 Maitreya Ghatak, 'Health and Nutrition', in Jasodhara Bagchi, ed. *The Changing Status of Women in West Bengal, 1970–2000: The Challenge Ahead*, New Delhi: Sage, 2005, 44.
15 Ibid.
16 C. Sathyamala, 'Women's Health Movement in Independent India', in Amiya K. Bagchi and Krishna Soman, eds. *Maladies, Preventives and Curatives: Debates in Public Health in India*, New Delhi: Tulika, 2005.

17 Imrana Qadeer, 'Reproductive Health: A Public Health Perspective', *Economic and Political Weekly*, Vol.33, No.41, 1998, 2675–2684.
18 Mira Sadgopal, 'Can Maternity Services Open Up to the Indigenous Traditions of Midwifery?', *Economic and Political Weekly*, Vol.44, No.16, 2009, 52–59.
19 Partha Chatterjee, 'Nationalist Resolution of the Women's Question', in Kumkum Sangari and Sudesh Vaid, eds. *Recasting Women: Essays in Indian Colonial History*, New Brunswick, NJ: Rutgers university Press, 1992, 251.

# Glossary

*Antahpur*   Inner quarters of the Bengali household inhabited by women.

*Antahpur Siksa*   Home tutoring.

*Anturghar*   The small room located in an isolated corner of the household where women spent the period of seclusion before and after the birth of a child.

*Autcowroy*   A ceremony performed on the eighth day of the birth of the child in the Hindu household where eight kinds of parched peas, rice and sweetmeats along with cowries were distributed amongst the children of the house and the neighbourhood.

*Bahir*   Outside world.

*Bas Bhaban*   Drawing room.

*Bhadralok*   Gentlemen or western-educated urban intelligentsia in nineteenth-century Bengal.

*Bhadramahila*   Gentlewomen. Female counterpart of the bhadralok.

*Bhandar Bhaban*   Kitchen.

*Bharat Mata*   Mother India.

*Bustee*   Slum.

*Chakri*   Job.

*Daktar*   Practitioners of western medicine.

*Daktari*   Western medical practice.

*Dal*   Lentils.

*Desiya*   Local.

*Dhais*   Traditional birth attendants.

*Dhatribidya*   The art of midwifery.

*Garbhadhan*   The act of consummation which also forms the first of the sixteen rituals of the Hindus.

*Garbhinir Paricharya*   Care of pregnant woman.

*Griha*   Home.

*Grihakatri*   Female head or mistress of the household.

*Grihini*   Females in charge of household management.

*Hariloot*   Vaishnava practice which observed a much shorter period of seclusion for pregnant women and declared the mother and the infant clean after a simple ceremony.

*Janani*   Mother.

*Jatikkhoy*   Deterioration of race.

*Jatiya Svasthya*   National health.

*Jhal*   Hot and spicy.

*Kaviraj*   Practitioners of Ayurveda medicine.

*Kulin*   Good family from the three upper castes of Brahmin, Vaidya and Kayastha.

*Lajja*   Shame.

*Madhyabitta Shreni*   Educated middle class.

*Mahila Samitis*   Women's organisations formed in Bengal from the late nineteenth century.

*Pechoyepawa*   Neonatal tetanus affecting infant immediately after birth and causing death in most cases.

*Purdah*   Literal meaning is curtain. It denotes the practice of seclusion of Indian women.

*Purdahnashin*   Women behind curtain/women in seclusion.

*Ramanir Kartabya*   Duties of a woman.

*Saadh*   Ceremony performed for feeding the pregnant woman delicacies of her choice few days prior to her delivery.

*Santan Palan*   Child rearing.

*Shajya Bhaban*   Bedroom.

*Shasthi*   Folk Goddess regarded as the protectress of children.

*Shastras*   Hindu scriptures written in Sanskrit language explaining religious and legal ideas that underscored the Hindu way of life.

*Sisu*   Infant.

*Sisu Palan*   Infant rearing.

*Sutikagriha*   Place or site of birth in a Bengali household.

*Sutikajor*   Puerperal fever.

*Svasthya*   Health.

*Svasthya Raksha*   Preservation of health.

*Thaap*   Fire.

*Thana*   Police station.

*Vhaat*   Cooked rice.

*Vidhata*   God.

*Zamindar*   Landowner.

*Zenana*   Secluded quarters of a respectable household inhabited by its women (same as Antahpur).

# References

## Primary sources

### National archives of India, New Delhi

Government of India, Proceedings of the:
—— Home Department (Public Branch)
—— Home Department (Medical Branch)
—— Foreign and Political Department (Political Branch)

### West Bengal State Archives (WBSA)

Government of Bengal, Proceedings of the:
—— General Department (Medical Branch)
—— General Department (Education Branch)
—— Municipal Department (Medical Branch)
—— Judicial Department (Medical Branch)
—— Local Self-Government (Medical Branch)
General Committee of the Fever Hospital and Municipal Improvements, Miscellaneous Evidences and Papers, Appendix.
Reports on Newspapers and Periodicals in Bengal, 1891.

### Government publications

Bengal Legislative Council Proceedings, 1930–1947.
Beverly, H. *Report: Census of Bengal, 1872*, Calcutta: Bengal Secretariat Press, 1872.
Bourdillon, J.A. *Report of the Census of Bengal, 1881*, Vol.1, Calcutta: Bengal Secretariat Press, 1883.
*Maternal Mortality in Childbirth in India: A Summary of the Investigations Conducted Under the Indian Research Fund Association, 1925*, Calcutta: Government of India Central Publication Branch, 1928.

Neal Edwards, M.I. *Report of an Enquiry into the Causes of Maternal Mortality in Calcutta*, Delhi, Government of India: Manager of Publications, 1940.

O'Malley, L.S.S. *Census of India, 1911, Volume VI: City of Calcutta, Part I*, Calcutta: Bengal Secretariat Book Depot, 1913.

*Report of the Health Survey and Development Committee*, Vols.1 and 2, Delhi, Government of India: Manager of Publications, 1946.

## Annual reports

Annual Report of the Bengal Health Welfare Committee (Indian Red Cross Society) for the Year 1936.

Annual Reports of the All India Institute of Hygiene and Public Health, Calcutta, 1934–1946.

Annual Reports of the All India Women's Conference, 1927–1947.

Annual Reports of the Medical Schools in Bengal, 1918–1940.

Annual Reports of the National Association for Supplying Medical Aid by Women to the Women of India, 1925–1945.

Annual Reports on the Working of the Medical College, Calcutta, 1938–1939.

Report of the Ramakrishna Mission: Sisumangal Pratisthan – A Maternity Hospital and Child Welfare Centre, for the Year 1939.

Reports of the Bengali Sanitary Board and the Chief Engineer, Public Health Department, 1925–1941.

Reports of the Health Officers of the Corporation, Calcutta, 1909–1947.

## Medical journals (English)

*The British Medical Journal* (1870–1930)

*Calcutta Medical Journal* (1910–47)

*Calcutta Medical Review* (1939–41)

*Canadian Journal of Public Health (1944)*

*The Indian Lancet* (1890–1900)

*The Indian Medical Gazette* (1860–1940)

*The Indian Medical Record* (1917–52)

*Journal of the Association of the Medical Women in India* (1908–60)

*Journal of the Indian Medical Association* (1930–47)

*The Medical Digest* (1938)

## Medical journals and health magazines (Bengali)

*Bishak Darpan* (1900–1910)

*Cikitsa Prakasa* (1909–20)

*Cikitsa Sammilani* (1880–1900)

*Svasthya* (1900–1920)

*Svasthya Samacara* (1912–20)

## Women's magazines (Bengali)

*Antahpur* (1900–1905)
*Bamabodhini Patrika* (1867–1921)
*Bangalakshmi* (1926–36)
*Bangamahila* (1875–80)
*Bharati* (1890–1920)
*Byabosa O Banijya* (1934)
*Mahila* (1897)
*Paricarika* (1882–1903)
*Sachitra Sisir* (1920–24)

## Other periodicals and newspapers

*Amrita Bazar Patrika* (1920–47)
*Calcutta Municipal Gazette* (1925–46)

## Bengali books and pamphlets (before 1947)

Balfour, M.I. *Bharater Desi Dhaider Janya Dhatrisiksa* (A Guide for Indian Midwives), Calcutta: Baptist Mission Press, 1922.

Bandopadhyaya, Harinarayan. *Strirogbidhayak* (The Diseases of Women – Medical and Surgical – With Special Reference to Indian Disease), Second Edition, Calcutta, 1896.

Basu, Upendranath. *Kolikata o Uhar Corporation*, Calcutta: Sri Gouranga Press, 1944.

Bhattacharya, Kalikinkar. *Prasava-Vijnana* (A Treatise on Obstetrics), Calcutta: U.N. Dhar & Co, 1936.

Biswas, Radha Raman. *Garbhini o Prasuti Cikitsa* (Treatment of Pregnant Woman and Infant), Calcutta: Walker Homeo Hall, 1938.

Chattopadhyay, Khirodaprosad. *Dhatribidya* (Art of Midwifery), Bhowanipur: Oriental Press, 1886.

Chowdhury, Jogendra Lal. *Adarsha Janani* (Ideal Mother), Calcutta: Swarna Press, 1927.

Das, Sundari Mohan. *Saral Dhatri-Siksa, Kumar Tantra o Stri-Rog* (A Treatise on Midwifery, Infant-Rearing and Female Diseases), Calcutta: Premananda Das and Jogananda Das, 1940.

Dasgupta, Harimohan, *Ayurveda Dhatrividya Samgraha* (A Compilation of Ayurvedic Midwifery), Berhampur, 1917.

Deb, Shib Chunder. *Sisu Palan* (Child Rearing), Serampore: Serampore Mission Press, 1857.

Devi, Anurupa. *Sisumangal* (Instruction in Child Welfare and Rearing of Children), Calcutta: Bodhoday Press, 1926.

Dhar, Sarachchandra. *Adarsha Janani* (Ideal Mother), Dhaka: Nagendrachandra Roy, 1914.

Ghosh, Kiranchandra. *Stri-Cikitsa* (A Treatise on the Diseases of Women and Gynaecology), Calcutta, 1922.

Ghosh, Kisorimohan. *Garbhini Cikitsa* (Homeopathic Treatment in Pregnancy), Deoghar: The Criterion, 1914.

Ghosh, Mahendranath. *Saudaminira Dhatrisiksa Evam Garbhini o Prasuti Cikitsa* (A Work on Midwifery and Homeopathic Gynaecology), Calcutta: The Author, 1909.

Khastagir, Annada Charan. *Manabjanmatattva, Dhatribidya, Nabaprasut Sisu o Strijatir Byadhisangraha* (A Treatise on the Science and Practice of Midwifery with Diseases of Children and Women), Second Edition, Calcutta: Girish Vidyaratna, 1878.

Mitra, Girindra Krishna. *Prasuti o Santan* (Mother and the Child), Calcutta: Bengal Publishing House, 1936.

Mukherji, Debendranath. *Khokar Ma* (The Baby's Mother: Hints to a Mother on the Feeding, Rearing and Diseases of Infants), Calcutta: Aryan Press, 1902.

Mukherji, Kali Bhushan. *Matri Mangal* (A Play on Child and Maternity Welfare), Calcutta: Bengal Government Press, 1925.

Mukhopadhaya, Gangaprasad. *Matrishiksa* (A Treatise on Childbirth and Infant Management), Calcutta: United Press, 1902.

Mukhopadhyaya, Jadunath. *Dhatrisiksha ebong prasutisikshaar thatkathopakathanchhale dhai ebong prasutidiger protiupadesh* (Educating the Midwife and the Pregnant Woman Written in the Form of Dialogue), Chinsurah: Chikitsabodak Press, 1875.

Rai, Binode Bihari. *Ayurved Mote Sisupalan* (Infant Rearing According to Ayurveda), Rajshahi: Binod Press, 1891.

Ray, Haranath. *Dhatri-Sikkha Samgraha* (Midwife's Vade-Mecum), Calcutta: Bengal Law Report Press, 1887.

Roy, Devendranath. *Garhasthya Svasthyarakha Ebong Sochitro Dhatrisiksha* (Domestic Hygiene and Guide to Bengali Midwives), Calcutta: S.K. Lahiri & Co, 1904.

Sarkar, Abhaykumar. *Prasuti Paricharya o Sisu Palan* (Treatment of the Pregnant Woman and Infant Rearing), Calcutta: The Calcutta Publishers, 1937.

Sengupta, Gourinath. *Sharirik Swathya Bidhan* (A Treatise on Physical Health), Calcutta: Sambad Sajjanranjan Press, 1862.

Sengupta, Nagendranath. *Sochitro Daktari Sikkha* (Medical Education with Pictoral Illustrations), Fourth Edition, Calcutta: Nagendra Printing Works, 1905.

Sinha, Nityanand, *Saphala Stri Cikitsa* (A Treatise on the Treatment of Diseases of Women), Audulbaria: Dr Dhirendranath Halder, 1915.

## English books published before 1947

Balfour, Margaret Ida and Young, Ruth. *The Work of Medical Women in India*, Oxford: Oxford University Press, 1929.

Bose, Shib Chunder. *The Hindoos as They Are: A Description of the Manners, Customs and Inner Life of Hindoo Society in Bengal*, Second Edition, Calcutta: Thacker, Spink & Co., 1883.

*Centenary of the Medical College Bengal*, Medical College Centenary Volume Sub-Committee, 1935.

Das, Kedarnath. *A Handbook of Obstetrics for Students in India*, London: Butterworth, 1914.

Das, Kedarnath. *A Text Book of Midwifery for Medical Schools and Colleges in India*, Second Edition, Calcutta: Thacker, Spink & Co, 1926.

Dey, Lal Behary. *Bengal Peasant Life*, London: Palgrave Macmillan, 1878.

Green-Armytage, V.B. *Tropical Midwifery: Labour Room Clinics*, Calcutta and Simla: Thacker, Spink & Co, 1928.

Krishna, Kumar Harendra. *A Lecture on Female Education in Bengal: Delivered at the Bethune Society*, Calcutta: Bengalee Press, 1863.

McCleary, G.F. *The Maternity and Child Welfare Movement*, London: P.S. King & Son Ltd, 1935.

Mitra, Subodh, ed. *Transactions of the Obstetric and Gynaecological Congress*, Calcutta, 1941.

Mukherji, U.N. *Hindus: A Dying Race*, Calcutta: M. Bannerjee, 1909.

Rajwade, Laxmibai. *Our Cause: A Symposium by Indian Women*, Allahabad: Kitabistan, 1938.

Urquhart, Margaret M. *Women of Bengal: A Study of the Hindu Pardanashins of Calcutta*, Second Edition, Calcutta: Association Press (YMCA), 1926.

Young, Ruth. *Ante Natal Work in India: A Handbook for Nurses, Midwives and Health Visitors*, Maternity and Child Welfare Bureau: Indian Red Cross Society, 1931.

## Secondary literature

Allender, Team. *Learning Femininity in Colonial India, 1820–1932*, Manchester: Manchester University Press, 2000.

Amin, Sonia Nishat, *The World of Muslim Women in Colonial Bengal, 1876–1939*, Leiden, New York and Koln: E.J. Brill, 1996.

Amrith, Sunil. 'Political Culture of Health in India: A Historical Perspective', *Economic and Political Weekly*, Vol.42, No.2, January 2007, pp. 114–121.

Anderson, Warwick. *Colonial Pathologies: American Tropical Medicine, Race and Hygiene in the Philippines*, Durham: Duke University Press, 2006.

Arney, W.R. *Power and the Profession of Obstetrics*, Chicago and London: Chicago University Press, 1982.

Arnold, David, ed. 'Medical Priorities and Practice in 19th British India', *South Asia Research*, Vol.5, No.2, November 1985, pp. 167–183.

———, ed. *Imperial Medicine and Indigenous Societies*, Manchester: Manchester University Press, 1988.

——— *Colonising the Body: State Medicine and Epidemic Disease in Nineteenth-Century India*, Berkeley and Los Angeles: University of California Press, 1993.

——— *Science, Technology and Medicine in Colonial India*, Cambridge: Cambridge University Press, 2000.

———— 'Official Attitudes to Population, Birth Control and Reproductive Health in India, 1921–1946', in Sarah Hodges, ed. *Reproductive Health in India: History, Politics, Controversies*, New Delhi: Orient Longman, 2006.

Arnold, David and Sarkar, Sumit. 'In Search of Rational Remedies: Homeopathy in 19th-Century Bengal', in Waltraud Ernst, ed. *Plural Medicine: Tradition and Modernity, 1800–2000*, London and New York: Rutledge, 2000.

Bagchi, Amiya and Soman, Krishna. eds. *Maladies, Preventives and Curatives: Debates in Public Health in India*, Kolkata: Tulika Books, 2005.

Bagchi, Jasodhara. 'Representing Nationalism: Ideology of Motherhood in Colonial Bengal', *Economic and Political Weekly*, Vol.25, Nos.42–43, October 1990, pp. 65–71.

Bala, Poonam. *Imperialism and Medicine: A Socio-Historical Perspective*, New Delhi: Sage Publications, 1991.

————, ed. *Contesting Colonial Authority: Medicine and Indigenous Responses in Nineteenth- and Twentieth Century India*, Plymouth: Lexington Books, 2012.

Bannerji, Himani. 'Fashioning a Self: Educational Proposals for and by Women in Popular Magazines in Colonial Bengal', *Economic and Political Weekly*, Vol.26, No.43, October 1991, WS56–WS60.

———— 'Projects of Hegemony: Towards a Critique of Subaltern Studies "Resolution of the Women's Question"', *Economy and Political Weekly*, Vol.35, No.11, March 2000, pp. 902–920.

Bashford, Alison and Levine, Philippa, eds. *The Oxford Handbook of the History of Eugenics*, New York: Oxford University Press, 2010.

Basu, Aparna and Ray, Bharati. *Women's Struggle: A History of the All India Women's Conference, 1927–2002*, New Delhi: Manohar, 2003.

Bhattacharya, Jayanta. 'Anatomical Knowledge and East-West Exchange', in Deepak Kumar and Raj Sekhar Basu, eds. *Medical Encounters in British India*, New Delhi: Oxford University Press, 2013.

———— 'The Genesis of Hospital Medicine in India: The Calcutta Medical College (CMC) and the Emergence of a New Medical Epistemology', in *Indian Economic and Social History Review*, April–June, 2014, pp. 231–264.

Bhattacharya, Malini and Sen, Abhijit, ed. *Talking of Power, Early Writings of Bengali Women*, New Delhi: Stree, 2003.

Borst, Charlotte. *Catching Babies: The Professionalisation of Childbirth, 1870–1920*, Cambridge: Harvard University Press, 1995.

Borthwick, Meredith. *The Changing Role of Women in Bengal, 1849–1905*, Princeton, NJ: Princeton University Press, 1984.

Bose, Pradip Kumar, ed. *Health and Society in Bengal: A Selection from Late 19th-Century Bengali Periodicals*, New Delhi: Sage, 2006.

Branca, Patricia. *Silent Sisterhood: Middle Class Women in the Victorian Home*, London: Croom Helm, 1978.

Broomfield, J.H. *Elite Conflict in a Plural Society: 20th Century Bengal*, Berkeley: California University Press, 1968.

Burton, Antoinette. 'Contesting the *Zenana*: The Mission to Make Lady Doctors for India, 1874–1885', *The Journal of British Studies*, Vol.35, No.3, 1996, pp. 368–397.

Chakrabarty, Dipesh. 'The Difference: Deferral of (A) Colonial Modernity: Public Debates on Domesticity in British Bengal', *History Workshop*, Vol.36, 1993, pp. 1–34.

Chakraborty, Rachana. 'Women's Education and Empowerment in Colonial Bengal', in Hans Hagerdal, ed. *Responding to the West: Essays on Colonial Agency and Asian Agency*, Amsterdam: Amsterdam University Press, 2009.

Chatterjee, Partha. *Nationalist Thought and the Colonial World: A Derivative Discourse*, Second Edition, London: Zed Books, 1993.

——— *Nation and Its Fragments: Colonial and Post-Colonial Histories*, New Delhi: Oxford University Press, 1997.

——— 'Our Modernity', in Partha Chatterjee, ed. *Empire and Nation: Selected Essays*, New York: Columbia University Press, 2010.

Chowdhury, Indira. *The Frail Hero and Virile History: Gender and the Politics of Culture in Colonial Bengal*, Delhi: Oxford University Press, 1998.

Das, Shinjini. 'Debating Scientific Medicine: Homeopathy and Allopathy in Late 19th-Century Medical Print in Bengal', *Medical History*, Vol.56, No.4, October 2012, pp. 463–480.

Davin, Anna. 'Imperialism and Motherhood', *History Workshop*, Vol.5, Spring 1978, pp. 9–65.

Donegan, Jane B. *Women and Men Midwives: Medicine, Morality and Misogyny in Early America*, New York: Greenwood, 1978.

Donner, Henrike. *Domestic Goddesses: Maternity, Globalisation and Middle-Class Identity in Contemporary India*, London: Ashgate, 2008.

Donnison, Jean. *Midwives and Medical Men: A History of the Struggle for the Control of Childbirth*, Second Edition, London: Historical Publications Ltd, 1988.

Dutta, Pradip Kumar. *Carving Blocs: Communal Ideology in Early 20th-Century Bengal*, New Delhi: Oxford University Press, 1999.

Engels, Dagmar. *Beyond Purdah? Women in Bengal, 1890–1930*, New Delhi: Oxford University Press, 1996.

Farley, John. *To Cast Out Disease: A History of the International Health Division of the Rockefeller Foundation (1913–1951)*, New York: Oxford University Press, 2004.

Forbes, Geraldine. 'Managing Midwifery in India', in D. Engels and Shula Marks, eds. *Contesting Colonial Hegemony: State and Society in Africa and India*, London: German Historical Institute, 1994.

——— 'Education to Earn: Training Women in the Medical Professions', in Geraldine Forbes, ed. *Women in Colonial India: Essays on Politics, Medicine, and Historiography*, New Delhi: Chronicle Books, 2005.

——— 'Medicine for Women: "Lady Doctors" in the Districts of Bengal', in Geraldine Forbes, ed. *Women in Colonial India: Essays on Politics, Medicine, and Historiography*, New Delhi: Chronicle Books, 2005.

Forbes, Geraldine and Ray, Chaudhuri Tapan, ed. *The Memoirs of Dr Haimabati Sen: From Child Widow to Lady Doctor*, Delhi: Roli Books, 2000.

Franda, Marcus F. 'West Bengal', in Myron Winer, ed. *State Politics in India*, Princeton, NJ: Princeton University Press, 1968.

Ghatak, Maitreya. 'Health and Nutrition', in Jasodhara Bagchi, ed. *The Changing Status of Women in West Bengal, 1970–2000: The Challenge Ahead*, New Delhi: Sage, 2005.

Ghose, Benoy. 'The Crisis of Bengali Gentility in Calcutta', *The Economic Weekly*, Vol.XI, Nos.26, 27 and 28, July 1957, pp. 821–826.

Ghosh, Anindita, 'Revisiting the "Bengal Renaissance": Literary Bengali and Low-Life Print in Colonial Calcutta', *Economic and Political Weekly*, Vol.37, No.2, 2002, pp. 19–25.

——— *Behind the Veil: Resistance, Women and the Everyday in Colonial South Asia*, Delhi: Permanent Black, 2007.

Gorman, Mel. 'Introduction of Western Science Into Colonial India: Role of the CMC', *Proceedings of the American Philosophical Society*, Vol.128, No.2, September 1988, pp. 276–298.

Green, Monica H. 'Gendering the History of Women's Healthcare', *Gender and History*, Vol.20, No.3, November 2008, pp. 487–518.

Guha, Ambalika. 'The "Masculine" Female: Women Doctors in Colonial India, c.1870–1940', *Social Scientist*, Vol.44, Nos.5–6, May–June 2016, pp. 49–64.

Guha, Ambalika, 'Beyond the Apparent: The Male Doctors and the medicalisation of childbirth in Bengal, 1840s-1940s', *Indian Historical Review*, Vol.44, No.1, June 2017, pp.1–18.

Guha, Supriya. 'From Dais to Doctors: The Medicalisation of Childbirth in Colonial India', in Lakhsmi Lingam, ed. *Understanding Women's Health Issues: A Reader*, New Delhi: Kali, 1998, pp. 145–162.

——— ' "The best Swadeshi": Reproductive Health in Bengal, 1840–1940', in Sarah Hodges, ed. *Reproductive Health in India: History, Politics, Controversies*, Delhi: Orient Longman, 2006.

Gupta, Charu. *Sexuality, Obscenity and Community: Women, Muslims and the Hindu Public in Colonial India*, New York: Palgrave Macmillan, 2002.

Harrison, Mark. *Public Health in British India: Anglo-Indian Preventive Medicine 1859–1914*, Cambridge: Cambridge University Press, 1994.

Headrick, Daniel R. *Tools of Empire: Technology and European Imperialism in the 19th Century*, Oxford: Oxford University Press, 1981.

Heimsath, Charles. 'The Origin and Enactment of the Indian Age of Consent Bill, 1891', *The Journal of Asian Studies*, Vol.21, No.4, 1962, pp. 491–504.

Hochmuth, Christian. 'Patterns of Medical Culture in Colonial Bengal, 1835–1880', *Bulletin of the History of Medicine*, Vol.80, No.1, Spring 2006, pp. 39–72.

Hollen, Van Cecilia. *Birth on the Threshold: Childbirth and Modernity in South India*, New Delhi: Zubaan, 2003.

Jaggi, O.P. *History of Science Technology and Medicine in India*, Delhi: Atma Ram, 1981.

Jayapalan, N. *Modern Governments and Constitutions*, Vol.II, New Delhi: Atlantic Publishers, 2002.

Jeffery, Roger. *The Politics of Health in India*, Berkeley, Los Angeles and London: University of California Press, 1988.

Jordan, Brigitte. 'Technology Transfer in Obstetrics: Theory and Practice in Developing Countries', Michigan State University, Working Paper 126, September 1986.

Jordanova, L.J. 'Natural Facts: A Historical Perspective on Science and Sexuality', in Carol P. MacCormack and Marilyn Strathern, ed. *Nature, Culture and Gender*, Cambridge: Cambridge University Press, 1980.

Karlekar, Malavika. 'Kadambini and the Bhadralok: Early Debates Over Women's Education in Bengal', *Economic and Political Weekly*, Vol.21, No.19, April 1986, pp. 25–31.

Kavadi, Shirish N. *The Rockefeller Foundation and Public Health in Colonial India 1916–1945: A Narrative History*, Pune and Mumbai: Foundation for Research in Community Health, 1999.

Kopf, David. *British Orientalism and the Bengal Renaissance: The Dynamics of Indian Modernisation 1773–1835*, Berkeley and Los Angeles: University of California Press, 1969.

———— *Brahmo Samaj and the Shaping of Modern Mind*, Princeton, NJ: Princeton University Press, 1979.

Kumar, Anil. *Medicine and the Raj: British Medical Policy 1835–1911*, New Delhi: Sage, 1998.

Kumar, Deepak. 'Calcutta: The Emergence of a Science City (1784–1856)', *Indian Journal of History of Science*, Vol.29, No.1, January–March, 1994.

———— *Science and the Raj, 1857–1905*, Delhi: Oxford University Press, 1995.

———— 'Medical Encounters in British India, 1820–1920', *Economic and Political Weekly*, Vol.32, No.4, January1997, pp. 166–170.

Kumar, Radha. *The History of Doing: An Illustrated Account of Movements for Women's Rights and Feminism in India, 1800–1900*, New Delhi: Zubaan, 1993.

Kundu, Nitai, 'The Case of Kolkata, India', in UN Habitat, ed. *Global Report on Human Settlements: The Challenge of Slums*, Part IV 'Summary of City Case Studies', London: Earthscan, 2003.

Lal, Maneesha. 'The Politics of Gender and Medicine in Colonial India: The Countess of Dufferin Fund, 1885–1888', *Bulletin of the History of Medicine*, Vol.68, 1994, pp. 29–66.

———— 'Purdah as Pathology: Gender and Circulation of Medical Knowledge in Colonial India', in Sarah Hodges, ed. *Reproductive Health in India: History, Politics, Controversies*, Delhi: Orient Longman, 2006.

Lang, Sean. 'Drop the Demon Dai: Maternal Mortality and the State in Colonial Madras, 1840–1875', *Social History of Medicine*, Vol.18, No.3, 2005, pp. 357–378.

—— 'Saving India Through Its Women', *History Today*, Vol.55, No.9, September 2009, pp. 46–51.

—— 'Colonial Compassion and Political Calculation: The Countess of Dufferin and Her Fund', in Poonam Bala, ed. *Contesting Colonial Authority: Medicine and Indigenous Responses in Nineteenth- and Twentieth Century India*, Plymouth: Lexington Books, 2012.

Leavitt, Judith Walzer. 'Birthing and Anaesthesia: The Debate Over Twilight Sleep', *Signs*, Vol.6, No.1, Autumn 1980, pp. 147–164.

Lewis Jane. *The Politics of Motherhood: Child and Maternal Welfare in England, 1900–1939*, London: Croom Helm, 1980.

Loudon, Irvine. *Medical Care and the General Practitioner, 1750–1850*, Oxford: Clarendon Press, 1986.

—— *Death in Childbirth: An International Study of Maternal Care and Maternal Mortality, 1800–1950*, Oxford: Clarendon Press, 1992.

MacLeod, Roy and Lewis, Milton eds. *Disease, Medicine and Empire: Perspectives on Western Medicine and the Experience of European Expansion*, London: Routledge, 1988.

Mani, Lata. *Contentious Traditions: The Debate on Sati in Colonial India*, Berkeley: University of California Press, 1998.

McGuire, John. *The Making of a Colonial Mind: A Quantitative Study of the Bhadralok in Calcutta, 1857–1885*, Canberra: Australian National University, 1983.

McTavish, Lianne. *Childbirth and the Display of Authority in Early Modern France*, Aldershot: Ashgate, 2005.

Misra, B.B. *The Indian Middle Classes: Their Growth in Modern Times*, London, New York and Bombay: Oxford University Press, 1961.

Mitchell, Juliet and Oakley, Ann. *The Rights and Wrongs of Women*, Middlesex: Penguin Books, 1976.

Morantz-Sanchez and Regina Markell. *Sympathy and Science: Women Physicians in American Medicine*, New York and Oxford: Oxford University Press, 1985.

Morehouse, Ward. *Science in India*, Bombay: Administrative Staff College of India, 1971.

Moscucci, Ornella. *The Science of Woman: Gynaecology and Gender in England, 1800–1929*, Cambridge: Cambridge University Press, 1990.

Mukharji, Projit Bihari. *Nationalising the Body: Medical Market, Print and Daktari Medicine*, London: Anthem Press, 2011.

Mukherjee, S.N. 'The Bhadraloks of Bengal', in Dipankar Gupta, ed. *Social Stratification*, Delhi: Oxford University Press, 1991.

Mukherjee, Sujata. 'Disciplining the Body? Health Care for Women and Children in Early 20th Century Bengal', in Deepak Kumar, ed. *Disease and Medicine in India: A Historical Overview*, New Delhi: Tulika, 2001.

Murshid Ghulam. *Reluctant Debutante: Response of Bengali Women to Modernisation, 1849–1905*, Rajshahi: Sahitya Samsad, 1985.

Nag, Moni. 'Impact of Social and Economic Development on Mortality: Comparative Study of Kerala and West Bengal', *Economic and Political Weekly*, Vol.18, Nos.19–21, May 1983, pp. 877–900.

Nandy, Ashish. *The Intimate Enemy: Loss and Recovery of Self Under Colonialism*, Delhi: Oxford University Press, 1988.

Nath, Shankarkumar. *Kolkata Medical Colleger Gorar Katha o Pundit Madhusudan Gupta*, Calcutta: Sahitya Sansad, 2014.

Oakley, Ann. *The Captured Womb: A History of the Medical Care of Pregnant Women*, Oxford: Basil Blackwell, 1984.

Papps Elaine. *Doctoring Childbirth and Regulating Midwifery in New Zealand: A Foucaldian Perspective*, Palmerstone North: Dunmore Press, 1997.

Porter, Dorothy and Porter, Roy. *Patient's Progress: Doctors and Doctoring in Eighteenth-Century England*, Stanford: Stanford University Press, 1989.

Porter, Roy. *Health for Sale: Quackery in England, 1660–1850*, New York: Manchester University Press, 1989.

——— *The Greatest Benefit to Mankind: A Medical History of Humanity from Antiquity to the Present*, London: HarperCollins, 1997.

Prakash Gyan. *Another Reason: Science and Imagination of Modern India*, Princeton, NJ: Princeton University Press, 1999.

Qadeer, Imrana. 'Reproductive Health: A Public Health Perspective', *Economic and Political Weekly*, Vol.33, No.41, 1998, pp. 2675–2684.

Raina, Dhruv and Irfan, Habib S. *Domesticating Modern Science: A Social History of Science and Culture in Colonial India*, New Delhi: Tulika Books, 2004.

Raj, Kapil, *Relocating Modern Science: Circulation and the Construction of Knowledge in South Asia and Europe, 1650–1900*, Houndmills and New York: Palgrave Macmillan, 2007.

Ramanna, Mridula. 'Indian Practitioners of Western Medicine: Grant Medical College, 1845–1885', *Radical Journal of Health*, Vol.1, 1995, pp. 116–135.

——— *Health Care in Bombay Presidency, 1896–1930*, Delhi: Primus Books, 2012.

Ramusack, Barbara M. 'Embattled Advocates: The Debate over Birth Control in India, 1920–1940', *Journal of Women's History*, Vol.1, No.2, 1989, pp. 34–64.

Rao, Mohan. *From Population Control to Reproductive Health: Malthusian Arithmetic*, New Delhi: Sage Publications, 2004.

Ray, Bharati. 'Women of Bengal, Transformation in Ideas and Ideals, 1900–1947', *Social Scientist*, Vol.19, Nos.5/6, 1991, pp. 3–23.

——— *Shekaler Nari Siksha: Bamabodhini Patrika (1270–1399)*, Calcutta University: Women's Studies Research Centre, 1998.

Ray, Kabita. *History of Public Health: Colonial Bengal, 1921–1947*, Calcutta: K.P. Bagchi, 1998.

Ray, Rajat Kanta, ed. *Mind Body and Society: Life and Mentality in Colonial Bengal*, Calcutta: Oxford University Press, 1995.

Rosselli, John. 'The Self-Image of Effeteness: Physical Education and Nationalism in 19th-Century Bengal', *Past and Present*, Vol. 86, February1980, pp. 121–148.

Roy, Manisha. *Bengali Women*, Chicago and London: Chicago University Press, 1975.

Sadgopal, Mira, 'Can Maternity Services Open Up to the Indigenous Traditions of Midwifery?', *Economic and Political Weekly*, Vol.44, No.16, 2009, pp. 52–59.

Sangari, Kumkum and Vaid, Sudesh, ed. *Recasting Women: Essays in Indian Colonial History*, New Brunswick, NJ: Rutgers University Press, 1990.

Sarkar, Sumit. *Writing Social History*, New Delhi: Oxford University Press, 1997.

——— *The Swadeshi Movement in Bengal, 1903–1908*, New Delhi: Permanent Black, 2010.

Sarkar, Tanika. 'Nationalist Iconography: Image of Women in 19th Century Bengali Literature', *Economic and Political Weekly*, Vol.22, No.47, November 1987, pp. 2011–2015.

——— *Hindu Wife, Hindu Nation*, New Delhi: Permanent Black, 2001.

Sekhawat, Samiksha. 'Feminising Empire: The Association of Medical Women in India and the Campaign to Found a Women's Medical Service', *Social Scientist*, Vol.41, Nos.5/6, 2013, pp. 65–81.

Selin, Helaine. *Encyclopaedia of the History of Science, Technology and Medicine in Non-Western Cultures*, Vol.I, The Netherlands: Kluwer Academic Publishers, 1997.

Sen, Amiya P. *Hindu Revivalism in Bengal, 1872–1905: Some Essays in Interpretation*, Delhi: Oxford University Press, 1993.

Sen, Krishna. 'Lessons in Self-Fashioning: "Bamabodhini Patrika" and the Education of Women in Colonial Bengal', *Victorian Periodicals Review*, Vol.37, No.2, The 19th Century Press in India, Summer 2004, pp. 176–191.

Sen, Samita. *Women and Labor in Late Colonial India: The Bengal Jute Industry*, Cambridge: Cambridge University Press, 1999.

Sen, S.N. *History of Freedom Movement in India, 1857–1947*, New Delhi: New Age International Publishers, 1997.

Sen, Srabani. 'The Asiatic Society and the Sciences in India, 1784–1947', in Uma Dasgupta, ed. *Science and Modern India: An Institutional History, c.1784–1947*, New Delhi: Centre for Studies in Civilisations, 2011.

Sen, Samita and Das, Anirban, eds. 'A History of the CMC and Hospital, 1835–1936', in Uma Dasgupta, ed. *Science and Modern India: An Institutional History, c.1784–1947*, New Delhi: Centre for Studies in Civilisations, 2011.

Sevea, Iqbal Singh, *The Political Philosophy of Muhammad Iqbal: Islam and Nationalism in Late Colonial India*, New York: Cambridge University Press, 2012.

Singh, Maina Chawla. *Gender, Religion and 'Heathen Lands': American Missionary Women in South Asia (1860–1940s)*, New York: Garland, 2000.

Singleton, Mark. 'Yoga, Eugenics and Spiritual Darwinism in the Early 20th Century', *International Journal of Hindu Studies*, Vol.11, No.2, August 2007, pp. 125–146.

Sinha, Mrinalini. *Colonial Masculinity: The 'Manly Englishman' and the 'effeminate Bengali' in the Late 19th Century*, Manchester and New York: Manchester University Press, 1995.

———— *Mother India: Selections from the Controversial 1927 Text*, Delhi: Kali for Women Press, 1998.

———— 'Gender in the Critiques of Colonialism and Nationalism: Locating the Indian Woman', in Tanika Sarkar and Sumit Sarkar, eds. *Women and Social Reform in Modern India: A Reader*, Indiana: Indiana University Press, 2008.

Smith, Philippa Mein. *Maternity in Dispute: New Zealand, 1920–1939*, Department of Internal Affairs: Historical Publications Branch, 1986.

Soman, Krishna. 'Women, Medicine and Politics of Gender: Institution of Traditional Midwives in 20th Century Bengal', Institute of Development Studies, Occasional Paper 32, November 2011.

Theriot, Nancy M. 'Women's Voices in Nineteenth-Century Medical Discourse: A Step Towards Deconstructing Science', *Signs*, Vol.19, No.1, Autumn 1993, pp. 1–31.

Viswanathan, Gauri. *Masks of Conquest: Literary Study and British Rule in India*, New York: Columbia University Press, 1989.

Walsh, Judith. 'The Virtuous Wife and the Well-Ordered Home: The Reconceptualization of Bengali Women and Their Worlds', in Rajat Kanta Ray, ed. *Mind, Body and Society: Life and Mentality in Colonial Bengal*, Calcutta: Oxford University Press, 1995.

Wilson, Adrian. *The Making of Man-Midwifery: Childbirth in England, 1660–1770*, London: UCL Press, 1995.

Wilson, Philip K., ed. *Childbirth: The Medicalisation of Obstetrics: Personnel, Practice and Instruments*, New York and London: Garland Publishing House, 1996.

Wood, Carl, ed. *Fifth World Congress of Gynaecology and Obstetrics*, Sydney: Butterworths, 1967.

## Unpublished PhD study

Guha, Supriya. 'A History of the Medicalisation of Childbirth in Bengal in the Late Nineteenth and Early Twentieth Centuries', Unpublished PhD dissertation, University of Calcutta, 1996.

Mitra, Samarpita. 'The Literary Public Sphere in Bengal: Aesthetics, Culture and Politics, 1905–1939', Unpublished PhD dissertation, University of Syracuse, 2009.

Paul, Chandrika. 'The Uneasy alliance: The Work of British and Bengali Medical Professionals, 1870–1935', Unpublished PhD dissertation, University of Cincinnati, 1997.

# Index